W9-CDB-813

theclinics.com

SURGICAL CLINICS OF NORTH AMERICA

Surgical Palliative Care

GUEST EDITOR
Geoffrey P. Dunn, MD, FACS

April 2005 • Volume 85 • Number 2

SAUNDERS

An Imprint of Elsevier, Inc.
PHILADELPHIA   LONDON   TORONTO   MONTREAL   SYDNEY   TOKYO

W.B. SAUNDERS COMPANY
A Division of Elsevier Inc.

1600 John F. Kennedy Blvd., Suite 1800, Philadelphia, PA 19103-2899

http://www.theclinics.com

SURGICAL CLINICS OF NORTH AMERICA
April 2005
Editor: Catherine Bewick

Volume 85, Number 2
ISSN 0039–6109
ISBN 1-4160-2791-2

Reprints. For copies of 100 or more of articles in this publication, please contact the commercial Reprints Department Elsevier Inc., 360 Park Avenue South, New York, New York 10010-1710. Tel. (212) 633-3813, Fax: (212) 462-1935, email: reprints@elsevier.com

The ideas and opinions expressed in *The Surgical Clinics of North America* do not necessarily reflect those of the Publisher. The Publisher does not assume any responsibility for any injury and/or damage to persons or property arising out of or related to any use of the material contained in this periodical. The reader is advised to check the appropriate medical literature and the product information currently provided by the manufacturer of each drug to be administered to verify the dosage, the method and duration of administration, or contraindications. It is the responsibility of the treating physician or other health care professional, relying on independent experience and knowledge of the patient, to determine drug dosages and the best treatment for the patient. Mention of any product in this issue should not be construed as endorsement by the contributors, editors, or the Publisher of the product or manufacturers' claims.

Surgical Clinics of North America (ISSN 0039–6109) is published bimonthly by Elsevier; Corporate and editorial Offices: 1600 John F. Kennedy Blvd., Suite 1800, Philadelphia, PA 19103-2899. Accounting and circulation offices: 6277 Sea Harbor Drive, Orlando, FL 32887-4800. Periodicals postage paid at Orlando, FL 32862, and additional mailing offices. Subscription prices are $190.00 per year for US individuals, $299.00 per year for US institutions, $95.00 per year for US students and residents, $234.00 per year for Canadian individuals, $365.00 per year for Canadian institutions, $250.00 for international individuals, $365.00 for international institutions and $125.00 per year for Canadian and foreign students/residents. To receive student/resident rate, orders must be accompanied by name of affiliated institution, date of term, and the *signature* of program/residency coordinator on institution letterhead. Orders will be billed at individual rate until proof of status is received. Foreign air speed delivery is included in all *Clinics* subscription prices. All prices are subject to change without notice. POSTMASTER: Send address changes to *The Surgical Clinics of North America*, W.B. Saunders Company, Periodicals Fulfillment, Orlando, FL 32887-4800. **Customer Service: 1-800-654-2452 (US). From outside of the US, call 1-407-345-1000.**

The Surgical Clinics of North America is also published in Spanish by McGraw-Hill Interamericana Editores S.A., P.O. Box 5-237 06500 Mexico D.F. Mexico; and in Portuguese by Interlivros Edicoes Ltda., Rua Comandante Coelho 1085, CEP 21250, Rio de Janeiro, Brazil; and in Greek by Paschalidis Medical Publications, Athens Greece.

The Surgical Clinics of North America is covered in *Index Medicus, EMBASE/Excerpta Medica, Current Contents/Clinical Medicine, Current Contents/Life Sciences, Science Citation Index,* and *ISI/BIOMED.*

Printed in the United States of America.

GUEST EDITOR

GEOFFREY P. DUNN, MD, FACS, Department of Surgery and Palliative Care Consultation Service, Hamot Medical Center, Erie, Pennsylvania

CONTRIBUTORS

JANET ABRAHM, MD, Co-Director, Palliative Care Programs, Dana Farber Cancer Institute; and Associate Professor, Medicine and Anesthesia, Harvard Medical School, Boston, Massachusetts

ALBERT J. ABOULAFIA, MD, FACS, Alvin & Lois Lapidus Cancer Institute, Sinai Hospital of Baltimore; Department of Orthopaedics, University of Maryland Medical Systems, Baltimore, Maryland

FRED G. BARKER II, MD, Associate Professor, Department of Surgery (Neurosurgery), Harvard Medical School, Boston, Massachusetts; Assistant Visiting Neurosurgeon, Massachusetts General Hospital, Boston, Massachusetts

MICHAEL A. CHOTI, MD, Division of Surgical Oncology, The Johns Hopkins University School of Medicine, Baltimore, Maryland

STEVEN A. CURLEY, MD, Professor of Surgery, Department of Surgical Oncology, The University of Texas M.D. Anderson Cancer Center, Houston, Texas

MELLAR P. DAVIS, MD, FCCP, Director of Research, The Harry R. Horvitz Center for Palliative Medicine, Cleveland Clinic Taussig Cancer Center, The Cleveland Clinic Foundation, Cleveland, Ohio

GEOFFREY P. DUNN, MD, FACS, Department of Surgery and Palliative Care Consultation Service, Hamot Medical Center, Erie, Pennsylvania

DANIEL B. HINSHAW, MD, FACS, Medical Director, Palliative Care Consult Team, VA Ann Arbor Healthcare System; Professor of Surgery, Department of Surgery, University of Michigan Medical School, Ann Arbor, Michigan

MICHAEL G. HOUSE, MD, Department of Surgery, The Johns Hopkins University School of Medicine, Baltimore, Maryland

JOAN L. HUFFMAN, MD, FACS, Clinical Assistant Professor, Department of Surgery, Temple University School of Medicine, Philadelphia, Pennsylvania; Trauma Surgeon/Surgical Critical Care Intensivist, Crozer-Chester Medical Center, Upland, Pennsylvania

RUTH L. LAGMAN, MD, MPH, Director of Clinical Services, The Harry R. Horvitz Center for Palliative Medicine, Cleveland Clinic Taussig Cancer Center, The Cleveland Clinic Foundation, Cleveland, Ohio

K. FRANCIS LEE, MD, FACS, Department of Surgery, Baystate Medical Center, Tufts University School of Medicine, Springfield, Massachusetts

SUSAN B. LeGRAND, MD, FACP, Director of Education, The Harry R. Horvitz Center for Palliative Medicine, Cleveland Clinic Taussig Cancer Center, The Cleveland Clinic Foundation, Cleveland, Ohio

STEVEN J. MENTZER, MD, Division of Thoracic Surgery, Department of Surgery, Brigham and Women's Hospital, Harvard Medical School, Boston, Massachusetts

ROBERT A. MILCH, MD, FACS, Clinical Professor of Surgery, State University at Buffalo, Buffalo, New York

ERNESTO P. MOLMENTI, MD, PhD, The Johns Hopkins University School of Medicine, Baltimore, Maryland

ANNE CHARLOTTE MOSENTHAL, MD, FACS, Chief, Division Surgical Critical Care, Associate Professor, Department of Surgery, New Jersey Medical School, University of Medicine & Dentistry of New Jersey, Newark, New Jersey

TIMOTHY M. PAWLIK, MD, MPH, Surgical Oncology Fellow, Department of Surgical Oncology, The University of Texas M.D. Anderson Cancer Center, Houston, Texas

EDGAR L. ROSS, MD, Director, Pain Management Center, Brigham and Women's Hospital; and Assistant Professor, Anesthesia, Harvard Medical School, Boston, Massachusetts

DENNIS O. SAGINI, MD, Howard University Hospital, Washington, DC

A. REED THOMPSON, MD, FACS, Associate Professor, Donald W. Reynolds Department of Geriatrics, University of Arkansas for Medical Sciences, Little Rock, Arkansas

DECLAN WALSH, MSc, FACP, FRCP (EDIN), Program Director, The Harry R. Horvitz Chair in Palliative Medicine, The Harry R. Horvitz Center for Palliative Medicine, Cleveland Clinic Taussig Cancer Center, The Cleveland Clinic Foundation, Cleveland, Ohio

JONATHAN J. WOLFE, PhD, RPh, Associate Professor, Department of Pharmacy Practice and Associate Dean for Development and Professional Affairs, College of Pharmacy, University of Arkansas for Medical Sciences, Little Rock, Arkansas

CONTENTS

persistent pain has not been a priority for surgeons; however, armed with a few basic principles of chronic pain management, surgeons can play an important role in the continued management of their patients. Sharpening pain assessment skills and considering nonpharmacologic and pharmacologic interventions are the keys to successful chronic pain management in surgical patients.

Pharmacologic therapy for neuropathic pain is based on an evolving understanding of its underlying mechanisms, and often requires a patient, methodical sequence of trials that include the "four As": analgesics, antidepressants, anticonvulsants, and antiarrhythmics. Critical for success is a willingness to stay engaged with the patient to evolve a mutually acceptable plan and goals of care with realistic outcomes that emphasize symptom control and maximization of function. This article provides a brief overview of neuropathic pain–its mechanisms and situations that a surgeon might encounter–and presents principles and recommendations for its primary pharmacologic management.

Individuals who have advanced disease often suffer from intractable symptoms. We discuss seven of the more common symptoms that are seen in this patient population. The causes of these symptoms often are varied and pathophysiology of each symptom may be complex. There are various therapeutic interventions, however, that can alleviate these symptoms. A thorough assessment and a thoughtful choice of pertinent diagnostic tests will lead to the most appropriate management.

Spiritual issues become a prominent part of the experience of the dying as they try to make sense of their suffering and find meaning at the end of life. Surgeons often are prepared poorly to address the spiritual needs of their patients, and as a result, sometimes miss important opportunities for relieving their patients' distress. This article explores the nature of spirituality and its relationship to religion, the intersection of suffering and spirituality, spiritual care of the dying, the surgeon and grief, the possibility of healing in death.

can play an important role in treating effusive disease of the pleura and pericardium. Minimally invasive surgical interventions, such as the use of video thoracoscopy, can relieve dyspnea effectively and improve the quality of life for patients who have end-stage thoracic disease.

Approximately 10% to 15% of all patients who have cancer will be diagnosed with brain metastases in the course of their illness, although the incidence in autopsy studies is greater. Most patients live less than a year after diagnosis of brain metastases; however, it probably is the specter of physical and mental disability during that time that is feared most by patients and families. Not all morbidity from brain metastases can be avoided or reversed, but aggressive local treatment is now known to benefit many patients who have one or a few brain metastases. These treatments (surgical resection or focused radiation) are the main subject of this article.

This article presents new and innovative aspects of palliative care for orthopaedic oncology patients. Patient-centered palliative care involves effective and empathetic communication between the physician and patient, with the ultimate goal of providing improved quality of life for individuals who have terminal illnesses. Orthopedic surgeons need to be supportive facilitators who inform patients of the available treatments, risks, and benefits and incorporate these treatments into the wishes of patients and their families.

Pancreatic cancer, with an annual incidence of approximately 28,000 cases, is the fourth leading cause of cancer-related mortality in men and women in the United States. Bile duct cancer is much less common, affecting only 2500 individuals each year. Even though most patients with pancreatic or bile duct cancer are not candidates for curative surgical resection because of early metastatic spread or extensive local tumor involvement, palliation of obstructive symptoms and pain remains a core component in the management of these diseases.

FORTHCOMING ISSUES

RECENT ISSUES

The Clinics are now available online!

www.theclinics.com

SURGICAL
CLINICS OF
NORTH AMERICA

ELSEVIER
SAUNDERS

Surg Clin N Am 85 (2005) xi

Dedication

We, the authors of this issue, would like to dedicate it to **F. Harold Kuschner, MD, FACS**. Dr. Kuschner is the ultimate role model for surgeons who care for those who suffer. During the Vietnam War he served as a flight surgeon. After his helicopter was downed by enemy fire, gravely wounding him, he became a prisoner of war (POW) for nearly 6 years. For the heroism that he showed while providing medical care to fellow POWs, he received the Silver Star, among numerous other decorations for gallantry.

Since the war he has taken leave from his private practice in ophthalmology to serve on medical missions to underserved areas.

This quote from a letter that he wrote eloquently bears witness to the surgeon's basic impulse to alleviate suffering: "As a young military flight surgeon in the 60s and 70s, unfortunately, I spent almost six years as a POW of the Viet Cong...first in the jungles of Vietnam, and then in the notorious prisons of Hanoi. I had no medicine or instruments and could only palliate the dying prisoners, by simply holding them in my arms. Twelve died that way, ten Americans, two West German nurses mistakenly captured. I hope that I was able to ease their suffering and help them to the other side."

doi:10.1016/j.suc.2005.01.023
surgical.theclinics.com

SURGICAL
CLINICS OF
NORTH AMERICA

ELSEVIER
SAUNDERS

Surg Clin N Am 85 (2005) xiii–xiv

Preface

Surgical Palliative Care

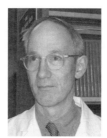

Geoffrey P. Dunn, MD, FACS
Guest Editor

The surgeon can expect to encounter a substantial number of patients who have progressive, incurable disease, as the primary physician and as a consultant.

This issue acknowledges that the surgeon may have cognitive and psychologic barriers to his or her own confidence in addressing the problems that are associated with chronic progressive or terminal illness. The issue is offered as a point of reference for surgeons of different specialties who are seeking guidance for management of the salient problems that are encountered in palliative care, which is care whose goal is to relieve suffering and improve quality of life in the context of an individual's family and society. The three pillars of palliative care are: (1) pain and nonpain symptom management; (2) communication between patients, families, and care providers; and (3) continuity of care across a range of clinical settings and services [1]. The indications for palliative care are based on the need for these services, not prognosis.

The first article introduces the historic and philosophical background of palliative care, addresses palliative care's current status in the field of surgery, and concludes by affirming it as a durable philosophy of surgical care that is applicable across a wide spectrum of illnesses. Following this are articles that cover basic palliative care skills, such as chronic pain management and palliative care assessment. Several articles have been included to introduce the general surgeon to surgical palliative care techniques and concepts in other surgical subspecialties, including transplantation, which usually is not associated with palliative care. The issue concludes with an article on the status of palliative care education for

doi:10.1016/j.suc.2005.01.024   *surgical.theclinics.com*

surgeons and surgeons-in-training. Although much of the material addresses oncologic illness, the principles and many of the interventions that are covered are clearly applicable to the much wider spectrum of illnesses.

Although the field of palliative care mostly has been developed by nonsurgeons, we face the same problems, and, in recent years, have begun to find our own collective voice in these matters. Palliative care challenges some of our most basic assumptions about the meaning of illness which leads us to ask new questions and discover new problems. As surgeons, we have a long tradition of service in the relief of suffering that precedes our recent accomplishments in eliminating disease. We can reclaim that tradition without compromising the bounty of life-saving innovation of the past half century. For a start, we must acknowledge the worthiness of a philosophy of care that represents a shift from elimination of disease to the unconditional relief of suffering and the affirmation of our patients' lives.

Geoffrey P. Dunn, MD, FACS
Department of Surgery and Palliative Care Consultation Service
Hamot Medical Center
201 State Street
Erie, PA 16550, USA

E-mail address: gpdunn1@earthlink.net

Reference

[1] Dunn GP. Restoring palliative care as a surgical tradition. Bull Am Coll Surg 2004;89(4):24.

ELSEVIER
SAUNDERS

Surg Clin N Am 85 (2005) 169–190

SURGICAL
CLINICS OF
NORTH AMERICA

Surgical Palliative Care: An Enduring Framework for Surgical Care

Geoffrey P. Dunn, MD, FACS

Department of Surgery and Palliative Care Consultation Service, Hamot Medical Center,
201 State Street, Erie, PA 16550, USA

During the past few years the field of surgery has joined others that recognize palliative care as an essential component of patient care [1]. For many surgeons, this recognition was accelerated by favorable personal experience with patients and relatives who had received hospice care or by haunting memories of patients whose illness and death had none of the redeeming qualities of comfort, dignity, or meaning. This growing awareness by surgeons has occurred against the background of the public's increasing expectations of improved end-of-life care, curiously juxtaposed with its obsession with curative or life-prolonging "breakthroughs." The medical care establishment and the cancer care establishment, in particular, seem to be going through "the five stages" of adaptation to the loss of the traditional biophysical model of disease management, starting in the stage of denial and gradually working its way to acceptance of a newer model that is centered on personhood, instead of disease.

In the 1980s we rarely saw the keywords "quality of life" in the medical literature, we rarely had discussions with patients and families who were anticipate irreversible decline that would trigger the designation of proxies and advanced directives, and we always felt awkward or powerless when our patients reached the point when irreversible physical decline was inevitable. Hospice referrals usually were late and reluctant. When the answers to our patients' physical problems ran out, there were no more answers, except, "there is no more we can do." Despite a generally brightening outlook for improved palliative care since then, patients still give distressing testimony to their sense of emotional abandonment by their treating physicians when their disease has progressed to the point of no further treatment [2]. During this interval of 20 years, much has happened to establish palliative care as a health philosophy that will improve the practice of surgery, conversely;

E-mail address: gpdunn1@earthlink.net

doi:10.1016/j.suc.2005.01.020   *surgical.theclinics.com*

much has happened in surgery that will improve palliative care. This synergy ultimately will encourage the application of this philosophy to a much broader spectrum of patients than those who traditionally have been associated with hospice care.

Historic and philosophic background of palliative care

There is little doubt that the art and science of palliative care had its origins in the modern hospice movement of which Dame Cicely Saunders was the salient pioneer. Much of the rapid and worldwide spread of the hospice concept, and subsequently, palliative care, can be traced to three specific contributions from her long and productive career. Her first major contribution, a clinical one, was her demonstration that terminally ill patients who suffered from cancer pain enjoyed improved quality of life with the scheduled giving of morphine. This was based on careful observations and meticulous record keeping at St. Joseph's Home during the 1950s in association with Howard Barrett, a surgeon, ironically, who eventually encouraged Saunders to study medicine. Saunders's discovery may be taken for granted now, but it has taken a half century for the scientific evidence, statutory change, and changes in societal attitudes to establish this as the standard of care [2a].

The term "palliative care" was coined by a surgeon, Balfour Mount, in the context of introducing the hospice concept to the Royal Victoria Hospital, an acute care multi-specialty hospital in Montreal. Surgeons were among his earliest and most steady referrers [2b,2c, see Table 1].

The association of hospice with palliative care has stigmatized palliative care for many health care professionals and lay persons who believe that palliative care is simply a semantic twist on "hospice," which they may have oversimplified already as "preparation for death." Hospice care can be classified as a subset of palliative care for patients in the last phases of illness. Downing et al [3] classified palliative care into three forms: active, comfort, and urgent, based on the degree of invasiveness and urgency (Box 1).

The physical model of medicine that is practiced in our death-denying, industrial culture has allowed death to remain the vanishing point of the human perspective. In contrast, a review of the historical evolution of hospice to palliative care demonstrates that both of these philosophies evolved as forms of social, psychologic, and spiritual health rehabilitation and maintenance that can occur in the face of ongoing physical decline. Doyle et al [4] states, "...palliative medicine is concerned with three things: the quality of life, the value of life, and the meaning of life." Seen in this light, it is existence, not death, that is the focus of palliative care. Threats to existence that correlate to suffering, such as occur in grave illness, inevitably provoke questioning from patients and caregivers about the meaning of existence.

Much of what is emerging in the practice and philosophy of palliative care has been influenced strongly by several models of suffering; suffering is the immediate target of palliative treatment. Complicating this orientation is the belief, in some cultures, of the positive and redemptive value of suffering. Although the willingness and ability to relieve suffering is the initial orientation of palliative caring, equally important affirmative qualities are identifiable, such as restoration and development of an individual's social, psychologic, and spiritual function.

Models of suffering

Several models of suffering emerged during the past 40 years that shaped the philosophy and practice of palliative care. An important influence on these constructs was the life and work of Victor Frankl. He was a concentration camp survivor who was a psychiatrist at the time of his captivity, and later, a progenitor of logotherapy, a form of existential analysis.

Frankl's [5] account of his experiences bears witness that survival is related to the capacity to make sense out of suffering, to give suffering a sense of meaning. The corollaries to this—and directly relevant to all palliative care—is that there must be a purpose to suffering and dying if one believes that there is any purpose to existence itself; choosing one's attitude in these situations is one freedom that cannot be taken away under any circumstances.

Frankl's life and work is a reminder of war's ironic capacity to stimulate innovation in the relief of human suffering. The Second World War and the hideous revelations in its aftermath followed this pattern, although far beyond the obvious examples of antibiotic therapy, blood banking, and burn care. Less obviously, the magnitude of this conflict's impact on the human condition is reflected 50 years later in the development of a healing philosophy that poses a fundamental challenge to the balance of power between doctor and patient, and the use of power itself.

The massive destruction of matter (atomic bomb) and the massive destruction of the soul (concentration camp) were two events that affected humanity's understanding of itself so profoundly that there is little wonder that all human undertakings, including the healing arts, have entered a period of skepticism and intensive self-reflection. This self-reflection has left us asking of ourselves, "When do we use our power and how do we live with the consequences of its use?". These questions, that result from developments in basic science of a century ago and geopolitics of the previous century, have found their way into the daily discourse of clinical care that is no longer satisfied with answers that were provided by the compartmentalized materialism that increasingly dominated science and medicine until the quantum era.

Frankl's experience addressed the relationship between suffering and existential issues. Since then, several concepts of suffering that were proposed by physicians have joined this discussion. In the early 1980s, just about a decade before significant social and legal debate about end-of-life topics that

Table 1
Schematic chart of Victoria classification of palliative care

Palliation type	Goal	Investigations	Treatments	Setting
Active (Blue)	To improve quality of life with possible prolongation of life by modification of underlying disease(s). Ex: Pt. who has potentially resectable pancreatic carcinoma. May require immediate symptom control or need guidance in setting future goals.	Active (eg, biopsy, invasive imaging, screenings)	Surgery, chemotherapy, radiation therapy, aggressive antibiotic use, Active treatment of complications (intubation, surgery)	In-patient facilities, including critical care units; Active office follow-up
Comfort (Green)	Symptom relief without modification of disease, usually indicated in terminally ill patients. Ex. Pt. who has unresectable pancreatic carcinoma, no longer a candidate for or no longer desires chemo or radiation therapy.	Minimal (eg, chest radiograph to rule out symptomatic effusion, serum calcium level to determine response to bisphosphonate therapy)	Opioids, major tranquilizers, anxiolytics, steroids, short-term cognitive and behavioral therapies, spiritual support, grief counseling, noninvasive treatment for complications	Home or homelike environment Brief in-patient or respite care admissions for symptom relief and respite for family

| Urgent (Yellow) | Rapid relief of overwhelming symptoms, mandatory if death is imminent. Shortened life may occur, but is not the intention of treatment (this must be clearly understood by patient or proxy). Ex. Patient who has advanced pancreatic carcinoma reporting uncontrolled pain (8 on a scale of 10), despite opioid therapy. | Only if absolutely necessary to guide immediate symptom control | Pharmacotherapy for pain, delirium, anxiety. Usually given intravenously or subcutaneously and in doses much higher than most physicians are accustomed to using. Deliberate sedation may need to be used and may need to be continued until time of death. | In-patient or home with continuous professional support and supervision |

Abbreviations: Ex, example; Pt, patient.

From Downing GM, Braithwaite DL, Wilde JM. Victoria BGY palliative care model—a new model for the 1990s. J Palliat care 1993;9(4):26–32; with permission.

Adapted from Storey P, Knight CF. UNIPAC 2: Alleviating psychological and spiritual pain in the terminally ill. Hospice and palliative care training for physicians. A self-study program. 2nd edition. Larchmont, New York: Mary Ann Liebert, Inc. Publishers; 2003. p. 24; with permission.

Box 1. Byock's four developmental tasks of the dying

- Renew a sense of personhood and meaning
- Bring closure to personal and community relationships
- Bring closure to worldly affairs
- Accept the finality of life and the transcendent

Adapted from Byock IR. The nature of suffering and the nature of opportunity at the end of life. Clin Geriatr Med 1996;12(2):237–52.

Adapted from Storey P, Knight CF. UNIPAC 2: Alleviating psychological and spiritual pain in the terminally ill. Hospice and palliative care training for physicians. A self-study program. 2nd edition. Larchmont, New York: Mary Ann Liebert, Inc. Publishers; 2003. p. 24; with permission.

---

primarily addressed patient autonomy, Cassell [6] pointed out in a landmark paper that when physicians deconstruct suffering to its physical dimension while ignoring the psychologic and spiritual pain that accompanies dying, they not only fail to relieve suffering, but compound it. He defined suffering as arising from the threat to integrity (wholeness) of the person [7]. He pointed out that "bodies do not suffer, only persons do." Persons are unique and experience disease differently. Persons suffer when their personhoods are threatened. The elements of personhood include the individual's past, present, and future; their social role; their private life; and a transcendent dimension. It is the presence of the person's transcendent dimension that permits the separation of death from failure. In Cassell's framework, suffering is not relieved until the threat to personhood has passed or is diminished.

The degree of suffering in Cassell's and other models correlates with the degree of existential threat. According to these models, intactness of personhood, not body, is the barometer of health. This conceptual framework resonates with the current popular interest in "holistic" health care and "treating the whole person." Although the public seems to be genuinely interested in the holistic model of health care and supports a multi-million dollar market for "alternative" medicine, the same public is an avid and generally contented consumer of health care that is organized according to the biophysical model. MacDonald [8] pointed out that the public never fully accepted the biophysical model of cancer because to most nonphysicians of all cultures, cancer always has been regarded as an illness with social, psychologic, and spiritual connotations. The biophysical model addresses physical threats to well-being or relies heavily on derivatives of it, such as pharmacology to address nonphysical problems. Translocating the goal of care from control of disease to ameliorating suffering inevitably will present our society with the same task of introspection that has been asked of physicians and surgeons to allow them to see "the whole person."

Dame Cicely Saunders's [9] model of "total pain" outlines four cardinal dimensions of pain (physical, social/economic, psychologic, spiritual) that contribute to suffering. Her theory brings a sharper clinical focus to Cassell's model of suffering by dissecting out specific areas where threats to personhood may lurk. It was more than coincidence that Saunders had previous professional experience as a nurse, social worker, and physician before her description of "total pain." Saunders's and Cassel's models could be seen, respectively, as the anatomy and physiology of palliative care. Brody [10] described suffering as the anguish felt by the individual as his life, a unique story, is fragmented which prevents its completion and transformation into a transcendent legacy. As the end of life draws nearer, the greater is the potential anguish. The implication for the surgeon is that patients who have progressive, life-limiting illness more likely may be seeking guidance in fixing their "broken stories" rather than fixing their broken bodies.

Perhaps one of the most positive conceptualizations of suffering and end-of-life is Byock's [11] view that dying is a natural phase of life that consists of a series of developmental tasks (see Box 1) with abundant opportunity for rewarding personal growth. His framework was one of several from this era that illustrates what previously had seemed so counterintuitive—dying could be conceived as the last phase of a succession of healthy activities, instead of a departure from health. The pragmatism of his model should appeal to surgeons who look for a yardstick by which they can gauge the relevance of specific therapies or the overall direction of care. The wide spectrum of these developmental tasks suggests that their applicability reaches much further back in the trajectory of an individual's life than the last phases of illness. This is particularly important for illnesses that are characterized by chronicity that is punctuated by life-threatening exacerbations that may initiate a prolonged period of overall decline.

In addition to the social, psychologic, and spiritual arguments that favor palliative care, there are economic reasons to consider substitution of a physical model of care (disease-directed therapy) with a palliative model sooner than the last 2 months of life. In an increasingly aging population, 28% of all Medicare costs are incurred in the last 2 years of life; half of this is spent during the last 2 months of life [12]. The Study to Understand Prognosis and Preference for Outcomes and Risks of Treatment (SUPPORT) [13] yielded abundant data to show that seriously ill hospitalized patients in the last 6 months of life, in addition to never getting better, frequently were undertreated for pain and their preferences for care often were unknown or even ignored. The average length of stay in hospice was 48 days; one third of patients died within 7 days. The difference between the total Medicare expenditures during the last 2 years of life, the increasingly shorter stay in hospice, and the incidence of failed symptom control that was identified in the SUPPORT study paints a picture that cries out for a model that is somewhere between traditional hospice care and curative care.

Palliative care and medical institutions

Kathleen Foley, a neurologist and preeminent proponent of pain management and palliative care, observed, "It is innately human to comfort and provide care to those suffering from cancer, particularly those close to death. Yet what seems self-evident at an individual, personal level has, by and large, not guided policy at the level of institutions in this country" [14].

The pace of institutional acceptance overall seems to be quickening in response to generous nonprofit funding initiatives and growing public awareness. Although palliative medicine was granted full medical specialty status in the United Kingdom in 1987 and the World Health Organization has endorsed palliative care in several statements since 1982 [15], institutional recognition outside of the hospice and palliative care organizations themselves has been slow in the United States. One of the first institutional endorsements was by the United States government. In 1982, the Tax Equity and Fiscal Responsibility Act established the Medicare Hospice Benefit (1983), less than 10 years after the establishment of the first hospice program in the United States. This was a legislative achievement that responded to popular pressure, not an initiative from any medical institution.

In 1996, the American Board of Internal Medicine published its education resource document, *Caring for the Dying*, specifically for the use of program directors and faculty of residency and subspecialty training. In 1997, the Institute of Medicine issued its report, *Approaching Death: Improving Care at the End of Life* [16]. This report concluded that suffering from serious pain and other burdensome symptoms, in many dying patients, has persisted despite the availability of effective treatments. A much needed remedy for this state of affairs followed in 1999 with the inauguration of the American Medical Association's sponsorship of the Robert Wood Johnson Foundation (RWJF)-funded EPEC project (Education for Physicians on End of Life Care). Since its initiation in 1999, EPEC has been used to train approximately a thousand physicians, including surgeons, to become instructors of other physicians and allied health care workers on the principles and practices of compassionate and competent palliative and end-of-life care. The concepts of palliative care are beginning to be taught in medical schools [17] and postgraduate curricula [18]. The number of articles that specifically address palliative care in the general medical literature has increased markedly since the time of the SUPPORT study in 1995.

Since 1996, The American Board of Hospice and Palliative Medicine (ABHPM) has offered its own physician certification examination, not affiliated with the American Board of Medical Specialties (ABMS). To date, roughly 1300 physicians have certified, including a small number of surgeons. The ABHPM is seeking, from the ABMS, added credential status for palliative and hospice medicine to those who are primarily certified in internal medicine and family medicine. At the time of this writing, there is no comparable arrangement for those primarily certified in surgery.

Palliative care and surgical institutions

The first official endorsement of the concept of palliative care by a surgical institution was the American College of Surgeons' (ACS) adoption of its *Statement of Principles Guiding Care at End of Life* in February 1998 [19]. The ACS's statement heralded surgeons' arrival to the robustly expanding field of palliative care in the United States at the end of the 1990s. Some surgeons recently proposed a more general revision of the *Statement of Principles* to reflect the wider spectrum of palliative care of which end-of-life care is only a subset [20].

In September 2001, the Promoting Excellence in End of Life Care National Program of the RWJF, in conjunction with the ACS, created a national Peer Workgroup to facilitate the introduction of the precepts and techniques of palliative care to surgical practice and education in the United States and Canada. The Workgroup brought together surgeons with demonstrated interest and background in palliative care with national leaders in palliative medicine. During the period of the RWJF grant, the Workgroup wrote a monthly series of articles about palliative care topics in the *Journal of the American College of Surgeons*, presented six symposia at ACS Clinical Congresses and Spring Meetings, established a website with the ACS, participated in the End-of-Life Education Project for Post-Graduate Training Programs, submitted questions for inclusion in Surgical Education and Self-Assessment Program 12, and wrote its *Report from the Field* [21], In October 2002, with the approval of the ACS Board of Regents, the Workgroup became the Task Force on Surgical Palliative Care in the College's Division of Education. The Task Force recently completed an instructional videotape on communication of bad news and it recently initiated work on an educational CD-ROM product.

In October 2003, the ACS' Task Force on Professionalism published the ACS' *Code of Professional Conduct* [22]. In their commentary, the Task Force wrote, "We singled out terminally ill patients as worthy of specific mention. Most surgeons are uncomfortable with death; it is an outcome that might be equated with defeat. Many surgeons are also uncomfortable with the transition from curative to palliative care. Effective palliation at these difficult times obligates sensitive discussion with patients and their families. Surgeons must accept a pivotal role in facilitating this therapeutic transition, for both patients and the health care team" [23].

Another important acknowledgment of the place of palliative care in surgical practice was the American Board of Surgery's inclusion in 2001 of palliative care as one of the domains in which the certified surgeon "... has acquired during training specialized knowledge and experience..." [24]. Since the late 1990s, the Royal College of Surgeons has had similar expectations for those sitting for its qualifying examination [25]. Palliative surgery and palliative care has been the focus of surveys and annual meetings of the Society of Critical Care Medicine and the Society of Surgical

Oncology in recent years. Fortunately, the increased awareness by surgeons of palliative and end-of-life care has occurred at a time when surgeons' attention has been increasingly directed to quality of life outcomes and their measurement.

Palliative care and quality of life measurement

Surgical institutions can do much to encourage the acceptance of quality of life (QOL) as a valid indicator of patient health through their participation in clinical trials. In any serious illness, questions that relate to surgical care's impact on survival and the nature of survival cannot avoid touching upon the hopes, fears, and other existential considerations of the individual. These subjective elements ultimately influence the individual's evaluation of the quality of his life. Because of the importance of the patient's perceptions in connecting the outer world intervention with the inner reality of the individual, the concepts of palliative care and QOL, although not synonymous, are inseparable. Strong arguments have been made for the scientific reliability of QOL measurement that should reassure skeptics in the surgical community that QOL outcomes measurement does not represent a "soft" standard, but the ultimate challenge to scientific ability, insight, and compassion [26].

Measurement of outcomes in surgical palliative care

QOL is the end point when measuring outcomes in palliative care. The twin goals of palliative care—symptom control and promotion of QOL—are not measured adequately by the traditional surgical outcomes measurements of mortality and morbidity. Finlayson and Eisenberg [27] identified three discrete definitions of "palliation" in the surgical literature that are, unfortunately, used interchangeably. These include: (1) surgery to relieve symptoms, knowing *a priori* that all tumor could not be removed; (2) surgery in which microscopic or gross disease was knowingly or unknowingly left behind; and (3) surgery for recurrent or persistent disease after primary treatment failure (ie, "salvage surgery"). These inconsistent definitions, often lumped together, make retrospective analysis of surgical literature highly suspect when evaluating surgical treatments for their efficacy for symptom control and promotion of QOL. Only the first of these definitions of palliation permits the patient to participate directly in the definition of success. The only one who can answer if palliation has been achieved is the patient.

Because patient report is the "gold standard" for measuring efficacy of palliative intervention, a new science of QOL measurement with psychometric validation is developing rapidly to fill this vacuum. Although the clinical outcomes movement may have been spurred by a wasteful health care system in the United States [28], it takes on an even greater moral purpose than cost containment when its momentum and prestige enhance the care of the suffering sick.

QOL measurements are based on patient questionnaires. Velanovitch [29] pointed out that QOL studies in the surgical literature generally have suffered from qualitative and methodologic deficiencies, although there is general agreement that QOL is a measurable construct. Rosenberg [30] argued that using functional assessment and QOL as bases for defining patient outcomes represents a needed philosophical shift from the traditional measurements of survival, morbidity, and laboratory parameters in patients who have primary malignant brain tumors. Sloan and Dueck [31] believe that educating the statistical community will do much to bridge the gap between investigators who want to assess QOL outcomes and institutions who want a sound scientific rationale and analysis plan for doing so.

QOL researchers generally agree that QOL measurement must embrace well-being and functional capacity in the psychologic, physical, and social domains. Some have added a fourth domain, the spiritual/existential, which is considered to be particularly relevant during the last stages of illness. Many of the most well-known and validated questionnaires do not address the spiritual domain specifically, although this element is likely to be added as a supplement to these. Spiritual/existential issues are assessed in some questionnaires that were designed specifically for palliative care settings, such as the McGill Quality of Life questionnaire (MQOL) [32]. The degree of emphasis on each domain and the number of domains that are assessed vary, although most of these instruments have been validated and some contain disease-specific modules. QOL questionnaires are self-administered. This poses some difficulties near the end of life when weakness, fatigability, and delirium limit the respondent's capacity to compete questionnaires. There is no consensus about the validity of proxy responses under these circumstances. Other problems in assessing QOL that are unique to the palliative care and end-of-life care setting include psychologic factors (denial, vulnerability) that influence symptom reporting.

The development of a QOL questionnaire, like palliative care itself, requires an interdisciplinary team approach. Identification of what is to be measured and how that will be determined by the choice of question list requires the participation of patients, medical practitioners, social workers, statisticians, and if possible, individuals with expertise in cultural and spiritual matters. Typically, prioritization and refinement of the questionnaire is tested in smaller pilot studies before larger scale validation studies that test validity, reliability, and sensitivity. Validity is a psychometric property that expresses the level of confidence that the researcher can have in the scores that are generated by the instrument (ie, validity determines the degree of relevance that a measurement has to what is being measured). Reliability is an indicator of the consistency of the scores.

Some commonly used validated QOL questionnaires include the Short-Form 36, European Organization for Research and Treatment of Cancer

Table 2
Selection of commonly used validated quality of life scales used in standard or palliative care settings

Questionnaire [ref]	Type	Items	Domains	Languages	Validation
Short Form 36 [33] SF-36	Generic Good for comparisons across populations and conditions or assessing patients who have more than one condition	36	• Symptoms • Physical • Social • Psychologic • Global QOL	Available in >40 languages Observer version available for family members and health care providers Short form available	Documented adequacy of psychometric properties Most widely used QOL instrument [34]
Functional Assessment of Cancer – General Version [35] FACT-G Updates: www.facit.org/ facit_questionnaire.htm	Disease specific Multiple diseases-specific modules	27	• Physical well-being • Social well-being • Psychologic well-being • Functional well-being	Available in 40 languages	Documented adequacy of psychometric properties
European Organization for Research and Treatment of Cancer Quality of Life Questionnaire-Core 30 [36] EORTC QLQ-C30 Updates: www.eortc.be/ home/qol/eortc	Disease specific Multiple disease specific modules	30	• Symptoms • Physical • Cognitive • Emotional • Social	Available in 38 languages	Psychometrics comparable to FACT-G [37]
McGill Quality of Life questionnaire [32] MQOL	Palliative Care Module developed for AIDS	17	• Physical symptoms • Physical well-being • Psychologic symptoms • Existential well-being • Support	Available in 7 languages (originally French and English)	Oncology outpatients Palliative care services Cross-cultural validation
Missoula-VITAS Quality of Life Index [38] MVQOLI Updates: www.dyingwell.org/ mvqoli	Palliative and hospice care	25	• Symptoms • Function • Interpersonal • Well-being • Spirituality	English, Spanish versions	Hospice

Quality of Life Questionnaire-Core 30, Functional Assessment of Cancer, Support Team Assessment Schedule, MQOL, and VITAS (Table 2). Different aspects of QOL are emphasized in these questionnaires which, to date, have shown low correlation. QOL assessments can be disease-, symptom-, domain- (eg, physical, psychologic), setting-, or culturally-specific, and many assessment tools use a modular design for specific applications with ongoing updates. When selecting a QOL assessment instrument, a surgeon is advised to select an existing validated tool from the hundreds that are available rather than initiating the lengthy and costly process of designing, testing, and validating a customized product. Information about specific instruments and peer-reviewed directories of instruments are available through the Internet.

Koller et al [39] argued persuasively that QOL in palliative surgical care can be addressed scientifically. Doing so, they postulate, should bring respect to the field that is necessary to encourage increasing participation by clinicians and researchers. They believe that these efforts ultimately would nudge public attitudes toward incurable illness, dying, and death in a more positive direction. Equally important for the conduct of palliative care, they note that the activity of QOL assessment is, in itself, therapeutic by helping to direct discussion of nonmedical issues that formerly were blind-sighted by a merely biophysical framework of discussion. This humanizing impact on patients and researchers by QOL research in clinical trials was noted by Sugarbaker et al [40], during the earliest days of the QOL concept in medical practice. That much has not changed since the early 1980s, although the medical world and society, in general, have changed in a way that allows QOL to share an equal place with survival as our highest priority goal of care.

Surgical palliative care emerging as a comprehensive philosophy

The dissonance of the existing surgical literature and the unevolved art and science of QOL measurement are not the only obstacles to the achievement of a durable philosophy of palliation for surgeons. The culture of mortality and morbidity rounds has presented a significant barrier to the acceptance of a philosophy of care that places equal emphasis on saving lives and the relief of suffering. In a symposium on surgical palliative care, oncologic surgeon, Cady et al [41] stated, "One of the basic principles of palliation, is that it is easier to make day-to-day surgical decisions in the framework of some overall surgical philosophy. Certainly if you have a mature surgical philosophy that understands the vicissitudes of life, you're better equipped to deal with some of these situations than a surgeon who thinks that 'I can cure all problems.'"

The association of death with failure or culpability poses the most profound psychologic barrier to the successful incorporation of a palliative philosophy into surgical practice. Closely related to this barrier are denial or fear of death, lack of training in the techniques of communication and symptom control, and in some cases, indifference. Other barriers to the acceptance of a comprehensive philosophy of palliation are deeply-rooted prejudices that are directed against the behavioral and social sciences (not to mention the humanities) as "less valid" than the physical sciences. Few of us can remember having been congratulated openly by our peers during "M and M" rounds for providing durable surgical symptom relief for a patient and solace to the patient's family, even if the reason for his listing on the mortality list was death due to underlying disease during the 30-day postoperative window. Even worse, the perception that "death equals failure" can become a disincentive for surgeons to "take on" patients who have end-stage disease for operative and nonoperative palliation.

The greatest conceptual and psychologic challenge for surgeons who wish to incorporate the enormous potential of palliative care into their practice is to understand palliation as an affirmative process of ameliorating suffering that takes an equal, if not greater, priority to the intent to cure.

Integrating palliative care into the practice of surgery: present and future

A survey of oncologic surgeons showed that palliative surgery is a significant part of practice—21% of their cancer operations were described as palliative in nature. In this survey, it also was determined that their previous education in palliative care was limited. Ninety percent reported receiving 10 hours or less of palliative care content in medical school, 79% reported 10 hours or less in residency or fellowship, and 74% reported 10 hours or less of continuing education in palliative care since completing their training [42]. One could extrapolate from this that nononcologic surgeons would be expected to have even less familiarity with palliative care because palliative and hospice care traditionally has been associated most often with oncologic illness. Despite the lack of formal education in palliative care, many surgeons recognize the palliative nature of much of their daily work.

Palliation through surgical care is more often a matter of rediscovery or renaming than assimilation of new concepts. The pragmatic temperament of surgeons facilitates their endorsement of any new technique or concept that effectively yields results—in this case, the relief of suffering. There is a wide spectrum of opportunity for the surgeon to participate in palliative care, depending on her time, abilities, and degree of interest. The decision of "How involved should I be in the palliative care of a patient?" is a personal one, but at the very least, the surgeon should be aware of the indications (Box 2) for referral and be willing to facilitate referral to the appropriate individuals or agencies in a timely and supportive manner. Years of faithful service by a surgeon can be forgotten quickly by a patient and family if there is foot-dragging by the surgeon about an appropriate hospice or palliative care referral.

Box 2. Indications for palliative care consultation

- Patient has an illness that is typified by progressive deterioration and worsening symptoms, often ending fatally.
- Patient has limiting/threatening conditions with declining functional status or mental or cognitive function.
- Suboptimal control of pain or other distressing symptoms.
- Patient/family would benefit from clarification of goals and plan of care, or resolution of ethical dilemmas.
- Patient/surrogate declines further invasive or curative procedures, preferring comfort-oriented symptom management only.
- Patients on medical/surgical or critical care units who are expected to die imminently or shortly following hospital discharge.
- Bereavement support of hospital workers, particularly after the death of a colleague.

Courtesy of Robert A. Milch, MD, FACS, Buffalo, NY.

For surgeons, there are several levels of involvement in palliative care beyond the primary level of engagement that is expected of all surgeons (Box 3). The full potential of a mature philosophy of palliation has yet to be realized in the management of numerous surgical illnesses [43].

The palliative care movement in the United States during the late 1990s and early 2000s has been catalyzed by the availability of several well-known websites. Among these is the End of Life/Palliative Education Resource Center (EPERC) website (www.eperc.mcw.edu) The purpose of EPERC is to share educational resource material among the community of health professional educators that is involved in palliative care education. The site offers "Fast Facts", peer-reviewed, one-page outlines of key information on important end-of-life clinical topics for end-of-life educators and clinicians (Box 4); educational materials that can be down-loaded; suggested articles; and, links to clinical and educational resource centers. The Center to Advance Palliative Care (CAPC) has a useful web site (www.capc.org) for surgeons who may be involved in organizing hospital-based palliative care programs. CAPC, a RWJF-supported initiative assisted by the Mount Sinai School of Medicine in New York, provides health care professionals with the tools, training, and technical assistance that are necessary to start and sustain successful palliative care programs in hospitals and other health care settings. Through its web site, management training seminars, audio conferences, and other offerings, CAPC provides a core curriculum for programs in planning

---

Box 3. Levels of involvement in surgical palliative care

Level 1

Surgeon is familiar with basic principles of palliative care as endorsed by surgical organizations and examining boards and has met palliative/end-of-life care continuing medical education requirements where mandated (California).

Surgeon is competent in management of acute and uncomplicated chronic pain, management of major nonpain symptoms, and communication of bad news.

Surgeon can recognize syndrome of imminent demise.

Surgeon refers appropriately to palliative care and hospice services.

Level 2

Level 1, plus...

Surgeon participates in palliative care indirectly or directly by participation in ethics, patient care, critical care, and pharmacy committees.

Surgeon promotes interest in palliative care by inviting grand rounds, supports educational initiatives, and supports palliative care consultants, services.

Level 3

Level 1, plus...

Surgeon, active or retired, participates in hospice or palliative care interdisciplinary teams either as paid staff or volunteer.

Surgeon is certified by AAHPM.

Level 4

Level 1, plus...

Surgeon is active in the practice of surgery whose primary focus is palliative care education, research, or surgery (surgical palliative care specialist).

Surgeon is certified by AAHPM.

---

and early stages of development. CAPC also provides information on palliative care to hospitals, clinicians, policymakers, payers, and researchers.

For those surgeons who wish to pursue palliative care in more depth, either as a primary focus of practice or as an adjunct to their primary specialization, there is the option of pursuing certification by the ABHPM. Candidates are required to hold an ABMS-approved Board Certification, certified status for at least 2 years in a primary medical specialty, have had 2 years practice experience beyond residency or fellowship, 2 years experience of interdisciplinary team work with a hospice or palliative care program,

---

Box 4. "Fast Fact" example from EPERC website

Fast Fact and Concept #003; Syndrome of Imminent Death
Author(s): Weissman, D.

Main Teaching Points:
1. Recognition
   Early stage: bed bound; loss of interest and ability to
      drink/eat; cognitive changes: either hypoactive or
      hyperactive delirium or increasing sleepiness.
   Mid stage: further decline in mental status—obtunded;
      "death rattle"—pooled oral secretions that are not
      cleared as a result of loss of swallowing reflex; fever
      is common.
   Late stage: coma, cool extremities, altered respiratory
      pattern—either fast or slow, fever is common; death.
*2. Time course: The time to traverse the various stages can be
   less than 24 hours or up to 10 to 14 days. Once entered, it is
   difficult to accurately predict the time course, which may
   cause considerable family distress, as death seems to
   "linger".*
3. Treatment:
   a) Once recognized, discuss with family, confirm treatment
      goals; write in progress note: "patient is dying", not
      "prognosis is poor."
   b) Discuss with family goal of stopping all treatments that
      are not contributing to comfort—pulse ox, IV hydration,
      antibiotics, finger sticks, etc. Hydration and feeding issues
      will need to be discussed sensitively, often eliciting more
      concern among the medical team than the family (future
      Fast Fact topic).
   c) Use Scopolamine patch (1 or 2) or Atropine to decrease
      oral secretions—"Death rattle".
   d) Use morphine to control dyspnea or tachypnea (it's very
      disturbing to families to see their loved one in a coma
      breathing 40/min (a goal should be to keep respiratory
      rate in range of 10–15).
   Note: this is not euthanasia! e) Opioids used to treat pain
      should not be stopped as death approaches—assume
      that the pain stimulus is still present; families always
      want reassurance that their loved one is
      not suffering.
   f) Provide excellent mouth and skin care.

Reference

Oxford Textbook of Palliative Medicine, 2nd ed. 1999, pages 982–9.

Fast Facts and Concepts are developed and distributed as part of the National Internal Medicine Residency Education project, funded by the Robert Wood Johnson Foundation.

DISCLAIMER CONCERNING MEDICAL INFORMATION Health care providers should exercise their own independent clinical judgment. Accordingly, the official prescribing information should be consulted before any product is used.

CONTACT Dr. David Weissman at weissmn@mcw.edu.

To find printer friendly Fast Facts, click on "Printer Friendly Version" located in the heading of each Fast Fact.

Copyright notice: Users are free to download and distribute Fast Facts for educational purposes only. Citation for referencing: Weissman, D. Fast Fact and Concepts #03: Syndrome of Imminent Death. June, 2000. End-of-Life Physician Education Resource Center www.eperc.mcw.edu.

Disclaimer: *Fast Facts* provide educational information, this information is not medical advice. Health care providers should exercise their own independent clinical judgment. Some *Fast Fact* information cites the use of a product in dosage, for an indication, or in a manner other than that recommended in the product labeling. Accordingly, the official prescribing information should be consulted before any such product is used.

Creation Date: 1/2000

Purpose: Instructional Aid

Audience(s)

Training: 3rd/4th Year Medical Students, Physicians in Practice

Specialty: Anesthesiology, Emergency Medicine, Family Medicine, General Internal Medicine, Geriatrics, Hematology/Oncology, Neurology, OB/GYN, Ophthalmology, Pulmonary/Critical Care, Pediatrics, Psychiatry, Surgery

Non-Physician: Nurses

ACGME Competencies: Medical knowledge, patient care

Keyword(s): Adult, Caring for families, Hydration, Negotiating treatment goals, Neurologic, Non-oral feeding, Oral/communication, Pain treatment, Prognosis, Skin/lymphatic

---

From Weissman D. Fast facts and concepts #03: syndrome of imminent death. End-of-Life Physician Resource Center. Available at http://www.eperc.mcw.edu; with permission.

physician and nonphysician professional references, and evidence of direct participation in the care of at least 50 terminally ill patients [44]. A small number of surgeons has been certified to date by the AAHPM.

The future of surgical palliative care research lies in the consensus of surgeons and their leadership that the concept of surgical palliative care is valid and essential to all practitioners. The conversion of rapidly fatal illnesses to chronic illnesses in an already aging population should provide some impetus to the acceptance of functional and QOL outcomes as equally valid as survival and disease-free intervals. The existing barriers to this are formidable and include economic and political obstacles, such as access to research funding. Only 0.9% of the 1999 National Cancer Institute budget went to palliative and hospice care research [45], despite the fact that a significant number of those persons who are diagnosed with cancer will succumb to it, still have it, or have permanent sequelae of its treatment at the time of death. The concept of surgical palliative care is still too new to identify research funding for nononcologic illness, such as peripheral vascular disease or transplantation. Other barriers include the unique ethical concerns that are related to research in a highly vulnerable population and little collaborative experience between surgeons and nonsurgical palliative care professionals. Promising surgical palliative care research can be identified in the younger generation of surgical oncologists, Krouse et al [46], McCahill et al [47], and Miner et al [37] in the US, and Easson et al [48] in Canada. They have addressed clinical surgical problems in the context of a comprehensive palliative philosophy to bring a much needed clarity and renewed luster to the word "palliate," in addition to developing a methodology for evaluating palliative outcomes.

Summary

Thomas R. Russell [49], Executive Director of the ACS pointed out in a recent editorial that the culture of surgery is changing and evolving, along with long-held values. He notes, "No longer is it 'my' patient, but it is 'our' patient." This shared responsibility for the surgical patient is not without peril, although this ethic has a positive application in the interdisciplinary model of palliative care. The principle of autonomy suggests that the patient, himself, shares some responsibility for a good QOL outcome. Although the focus of his remarks is fundamental change in residency training, his comments apply equally to the norms of surgical practice, especially palliative care: "We can start by building a sense of mutual respect for the broad range of individuals [including the patient and his family] involved in the care of our surgical patients, from nurses to allied health care professionals, from anesthesiologists to environmental service workers. As surgeons we must improve our communication and leadership skills, so these individuals will view us in a more positive light." Surgical palliative care is a philosophy of care that can answer this challenge.

Surgeons have always been up to the challenges of their era. They never have disappointed those whom they serve in their degree of courage, practicality, and innovation, but the changing landscape of illness and culture offer new opportunities for other insights and strengths to emerge.

References

[1] Cassel C, Foley K. Principles for care at the end of life: An emerging consensus among the specialties of medicine. Report sponsored by the Milbank Memorial Fund. December, 1999. Available at http://www.milbank.org. Accessed February 12, 2005.

[2] Brody JE. A doctor's duty, when death is inevitable. The New York Times; Tuesday, August 10, 2004. Section E, p. 7.

[2a] Jacox A, Carr DB, Payne R, et al. Management of cancer pain. Clinical practice guideline No. 9. Rockville, MD: Agency for Health Care Policy and Research, U.S. Department of Health and Human Services, Public Health Service; AHCPR Publication N. 94-0592: March 1994: 1–257.

[2b] Dunn G. The surgeon and palliative care: an evolving perspective. Surgical Oncology Clinics of North America 2001;10(1):7–24.

[2c] Ajemian I, Mount BM, editors. The R.V.H. manual on palliative/hospice care. New York: Arno Press. 1980;372–3.

[3] Downing GM, Braithwaite DL, Wilde JM, et al. Victoria BGY palliative care model—a new model for the 1990s. J Palliat Care 1993;9(4):26–32.

[4] Doyle D, Hanks G, Cherny NI, et al. Introduction. In: Doyle D, Hanks G, Cherny NI, et al, editors. Oxford textbook of palliative medicine. 3rd edition. Oxford (UK): Oxford University Press; 2004. p. 4.

[5] Frankl VE. Man's search for meaning. New York: Washington Square Press; 1985.

[6] Cassell EJ. The nature of suffering and the goals of medicine. N Engl J Med 1982;306(11): 639–45.

[7] Cassell EJ. The nature of suffering and the goals of medicine. New York: Oxford University Press; 1991.

[8] MacDonald N. Palliative medicine and modern cancer care. In: Doyle D, Hanks G, Cherny NI, et al, editors. Oxford textbook of palliative medicine. 3rd edition. Oxford (UK): Oxford University Press; 2004. p. 24–42.

[9] Saunders CM. The challenge of terminal care. In: Symington T, Carter RL, editors. Scientific foundations of oncology. London: Heinemann; 1976. p. 673–9.

[10] Brody H. My story is broken; can you help me fix it? Medical ethics and joint construction of narrative. Lit Med 1994;13(1):79–92.

[11] Byock IR. The nature of suffering and the nature of opportunity at the end of life. Clin Geriatr Med 1996;12(2):237–52.

[12] National Hospice Organization. Hospice fact sheet. Arlington (Va): National Hospice Organization; 2001.

[13] The SUPPORT Clinical Investigators. A controlled trial to improve care for seriously ill hospitalized patients. The study to understand prognoses and preferences for outcomes and risks of treatments (SUPPORT). JAMA 1995;274(20):1591–8.

[14] Foley KM. Preface. In: Foley KM, Gelband H, editors. Improving palliative care for cancer-summary and recommendations. Institute of Medicine and National Research Council. Washington DC: National Academy Press; 2001. p. ix.

[15] World Health Organization. Cancer pain relief and palliative care. Technical Report Series 804. Geneva (Switzerland): World Health Organization; 1990.

[16] American Board of Internal Medicine Committee on Evaluation of Clinical Competence. Caring for the dying. Identification and promotion of physician competency. Educational Resource Document. Philadelphia: American Board of Internal Medicine; 1996. p. 1–100.

[17] Billings JA, Block S. Palliative care in undergraduate medical education: status report and future directions. JAMA 1997;278(9):233–8.

[18] Weissman DE, Mullan PB, Ambuel B, et al. End-of-life curriculum reform: outcomes and impact in a follow-up study of internal medicine residency programs. J Palliat Med 2002;5(4): 497–506.

[19] American College of Surgeons. Principles guiding care at end of life. Bull Am Coll Surg 1998; 83:46.

[20] Krouse RS, Jonasson O, Milch RA, et al. An evolving strategy for surgical care. J Am Coll Surg 2004;198(1):149–55.

[21] Surgeons' Palliative Care Workgroup. Report from the field. J Am Coll Surg 2003;197(4): 661–86.

[22] American College of Surgeons Task Force on Professionalism. Code of professional conduct. J Am Coll Surg 2003;197(4):603–4.

[23] American College of Surgeons Task Force on Professionalism. Professionalism in surgery. J Am Coll Surg 2003;197(4):605–8.

[24] American Board of Surgery, Inc. Booklet of Information. July 2001–June 2002. Philadelphia: American Board of Surgery; 2001.

[25] Kirk RM, Mansfield AO, Cochrane JPS, editors. Clinical surgery in general. Royal College of Surgeons. 3rd edition. London: Churchill-Livingstone; 1999.

[26] Koller M, Nies C, Lorenz W. Quality of life issues in palliative surgery. In: Dunn GP, Johnson AG, editors. Surgical palliative care. Oxford (UK): Oxford University Press; 2004. p. 94–111.

[27] Finlayson CA, Eisenberg BL. Palliative pelvic exenteration: patient selection and results. Oncology 1996;10(4):479–84.

[28] Relman AS. Assessment and accountability. The third revolution in medical care. N Engl J Med 1988;319:1220–2.

[29] Velanovitch V. Quality of life studies in general surgical journals. J Am Coll Surg 2001; 193(3):288–96.

[30] Rosenberg J. How well are we doing in caring for the patient with primary malignant brain tumor? Are we measuring the outcomes that truly matter? A commentary. Neurosurg Focus 1998;4(6). Available at: www.aans.org. Accessed on February 12, 2005.

[31] Sloan JA, Dueck A. Issues for statisticians in conducting analyses and translating results for quality of life end points in clinical trials. J Biopharm Stat 2004;14(1):73–96.

[32] Cohen SR, Mount BM, Strobel MG, et al. The McGill quality of life questionnaire: a measure of quality of life appropriate for people with advanced disease. A preliminary study of validity and acceptability. Palliat Med 1995;9:207–19.

[33] Ware JE Jr, Sherbourne CD. The MOS 36-item short-form health survey (SF-36). I. Conceptual framework and item selection. Med Care 1992;30:473–83.

[34] Stewart AL, Ware JE Jr. Measuring functioning and well-being. The medical outcomes study approach. Durham (NC): Duke University Press; 1992.

[35] Cella DF, Tulsky DS, Gray G, et al. The functional assessment of cancer therapy scale; development and validation of the general measure. J Clin Oncol 1993;11:570–9.

[36] Aronson NK, et al. The European Organization for Research and Treatment of Cancer QLQ-C30: A quality-of-life instrument for use in international clinical trials in oncology. J Natl Cancer Inst 1993;85:365–76.

[37] Miner TJ, Brennan MF, Jaques DP. A prospective, symptom related, outcomes analysis of 1022 palliative procedures for advanced cancer. Ann Surg 2004;240(4):719–26 [discussion 726–7].

[38] Byock IR, Merriman MP. Measuring quality of life for patients with terminal illness: the Missoula-VITAS quality of life index. Palliat Med 1998;12:231–44.

[39] Koller M, Nies C, Lorenz W. Quality of life issues in palliative surgery. In: Dunn GP, Johnson AG, editors. Surgical palliative care. Oxford (UK): Oxford University Press; 2004. p. 94–111.

[40] Sugarbaker PH, Barofsky I, Rosenberg SA, et al. Quality of life assessment in extremity sarcoma trials. Surgery 1982;91:17–23.
[41] Cady B, Easson AE, Aboulafia AJ, et al. Part 1: Surgical palliation of advanced illness—what's new, what's helpful. J Am Coll Surg 2005;200(1):115–27.
[42] McCahill LE, Krouse R, Chu D, et al. Indications and use of palliative surgery-results of Society of Surgical Oncology survey. Ann Surg Oncol 2002;9(1):104–12.
[43] Dunn GP. The surgeon and palliative medicine: new horizons. J Palliat Med 1998;1(3): 214–9.
[44] American Board of Hospice and Palliative Medicine. Application handbook. November 2004 Examination. Available at: www.abhpm.org. Accessed February 12, 2005.
[45] Foley KM. Improving palliative care for cancer- summary and recommendations (eds. KM Foley and H. Gelband). National Cancer Policy Board, Institute of Medicine and National Research Council. Washington DC: National Academy Press; 2001.
[46] Krouse RS, Rosenfeld KE, Grant M, et al. Palliative care research: issues and opportunities [editorial]. Cancer Epidemiol Biomarkers Prev 2004;13(3):337–9.
[47] McCahill LE, Smith DD, Borneman T, et al. A prospective evaluation of palliative outcomes for surgery of advanced malignancies. Ann Surg Oncol 2003;10(6):654–63.
[48] Easson AM, Crosby JA, Librach SL. Discussion of death and dying in surgical textbooks. Am J Surg 2001;182(1):34–9.
[49] Russell TR. From my perspective. Bull Am Coll Surg 2004;89(12):3–4.

SURGICAL
CLINICS OF
NORTH AMERICA

Surg Clin N Am 85 (2005) 191–207

Preparation of the Patient for Palliative Procedures

Edgar L. Ross, MD[a,b,*], Janet Abrahm, MD[b,c]

[a]*Brigham and Women's Hospital, Pain Management Center,*
850 Boylston Street, Suite 320, Boston, MA 02467, USA
[b]*Department of Anesthesia, Harvard Medical School, Boston, MA, USA*
[c]*Palliative Care Programs, Dana Farber Cancer Institute, 44 Biney Street Southwest*
420, Boston, MA 02115, USA

Palliative surgery is used often to treat intractable symptoms. This approach to symptom management relies on a different premise than the usual goal of an invasive procedure. Surgical procedures traditionally have been used for diagnosis and treatment of disease, whereas palliative surgical procedures have been considered when the goal of curing was no longer possible, but a patient's symptoms suggested that an intervention was needed [1–4].

Preparation of the patient for palliative procedures

Well-planned palliative surgery is no less important for patient care than the traditional surgical goals of diagnosing or curing patients of their illnesses [2–4]. The differences between curative and palliative surgical approaches are presented in Table 1 [3]. Although the objectives may be substantially different, the two approaches are not incompatible and, in fact, can enhance each other.

Appropriate goals of any palliative procedure include pain and other symptom management, improvement of the patient's and family's well-being, assistance with the activities of daily living, and preserving the individual's function when possible. Palliative surgical procedures cross many different specialty boundaries, including all of the surgical subspecialties, anesthesia, interventional radiology, radiation therapy, medical oncology,

---

* Corresponding author. Brigham and Women's Pain Management Center, 850 Boylston Street, Suite 320, Boston, MA 02467.
E-mail address: elross@partners.org (E.L. Ross).

0039-6109/05/$ - see front matter © 2005 Elsevier Inc. All rights reserved.
doi:10.1016/j.suc.2004.12.005   *surgical.theclinics.com*

Table 1
Differences between disease- and symptom-oriented surgical care

Disease-oriented surgery: biophysical approach	Symptom-oriented surgery: person-centered approach
Cure or life prolongation is the goal	Symptom control is the goal
Analytical and rational approach	Subjective approach often used
Diagnostic-based	Symptom based
Based on scientific and biomedical approaches	Frequent reliance on humanistic and personal approaches as part of treatment planning
Treatment focused on disease processes	Efficacy of treatment not necessarily dependant on impact to underlying disease
Patient viewed as a set of organ systems and subsystems	Holistic care
Evidence-based medicine is the sole construct	In addition to evidence-based medicine, uses social science models
Can result in impersonal care	Treatment goals are individualized
Hierarchical care-providing, patient's role passive, and/or disease determines relevance of treatment	Frequently interdisciplinary, patient's role is active, and/or patient determines relevance of treatment
Death equates failure: *bad* or *tragic*	Death is natural/neutral: *sad*

specialties with endoscopic expertise, pain management specialties, and physical and occupational therapy.

This complexity requires an interdisciplinary attitude and management team to assure appropriate assessment and preparation of a patient for palliative surgery. In addition to evolving palliative care approaches, new organizational approaches are required to provide optimal care. This evolution is illustrated in Fig. 1. Until recently, concerns about the quality of life for a patient who had a life-limiting illness were only considered during the last stages of life. Little thought was given to the effects of progressing disease or its treatment on the patient and family. Palliative surgery usually was equated with giving up on a cure and often suggested that death was imminent. This misunderstanding frequently led to needless suffering; misperceptions about palliative surgery continue today.

Surgical palliative care is not the same as end-of-life care. The evolution of palliative care is shown (see Fig. 1). The first step or "old approach" in the evolution of palliative surgery was the consideration of palliative intervention only when the patient showed an urgent need for symptom control. No anticipation of other needs in the greater context was considered; a palliative care team (if available) only was consulted for selected areas of symptom management when these were identified. The second step in this evolution acknowledges that a patient could require palliative approaches to his illness at any point along the trajectory of his disease. This clearly is an improvement; however, the main drawback to this approach is that palliative care still is not included in the treatment process.

Evolution of palliative care

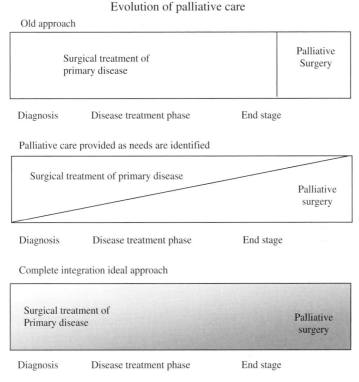

Fig. 1. Evolution of palliative care.

Waiting until identification of patient distress has resulted in an unfortunate underuse of effective surgical palliation and overuse of alternatives that are less effective. The third step in the evolution of the palliative approach completely integrates the domains of surgery and palliative care. This approach assumes prospective planning that leads to outcomes that are specific to a patient's/family's needs. This third approach is considered to be the optimal approach for surgical palliative care.

The assessment of a potential candidate for palliative surgical care requires a methodical approach and attention to detail [1,5,6]. The early and effective rapport with the patient, the primary caregiver, and the extended family is of primary importance to ultimate success. A positive report of a symptom from a checklist does not imply necessarily that the symptom is distressing or needs treatment. A problem-focused work-up should be comprehensive, yet be paced so that the patient does not become physically, psychologically, socially, or spiritually burdened. Repeated visits often are needed to complete the initial assessment. When treatment of the primary disease no longer is a feasible option, diagnostics should be limited to what would be pertinent to planning the palliative procedure. Pain often can be the limiting factor in the evaluation of the patient. A comprehensive assessment that uses a team approach can minimize discomfort by preventing duplicative procedures.

Because life expectancy can be limited for patients who are referred for palliative procedures, the primary treatment consideration should be lessening the patient's symptoms as much as possible while minimizing time and morbidity of recovery [7]. Even in the earliest stages of a patient's clinical course, the patient's needs during later stages of the illness should be anticipated. The assessment for palliative surgery is a four-step process, which includes: (1) patient factors, (2) what is feasible and what is possible, (3) psychosocial factors, and (4) available health care resources [8].

Patient factors

An in-depth understanding of patient factors requires a comprehensive assessment that determines the present health state of the patient, prognosis and natural history of a patient's disease, and identification of relevant symptoms of the disease process. Close collaboration with the patient's primary treatment team can provide a significant insight into a patient's disease course, past reaction to treatment, and the ability to be compliant with treatment plans [9]. Rapid advances in treatment have altered the natural history of many fatal disease processes significantly [1]. This is particularly true for oncology, but also is evident in the treatment of HIV and congestive heart failure.

Treatment should aim to provide durable relief for the anticipated time of survival. For example, a colostomy or colonic stent may be safer, faster, and equally effective for relief of malignant bowel obstruction than a resection and anastomosis. A patient who has a prognosis of many months with malignant ureteral obstruction would want to consider a ureteral stent rather than nephrostomy drainage, which would be more appropriate for a patient who has a shorter prognosis or more limited goals. Anticipation of a disease process also may lead to prophylactic procedures, such as stabilization of a weight-bearing long bone in a patient who has impending pathologic fracture. Prophylactic procedures that anticipate potential catastrophic events are important because of the greater complication rate that is associated with emergency surgery. Ensuring a tissue diagnosis and accurate disease staging is as relevant to palliative surgical planning as it is to surgery for cure, because this information can limit the scope of the operation that is necessary to accomplish the goal of symptom relief.

Preparation for palliative procedure can be facilitated by the categorization of a patient's symptoms into those that cause local, regional effects or generalized distress [10,11]. Only pathology-causing symptoms are relevant to palliative treatment. Examples of locally distressing pathology are nonradiating pain from metastatic disease to a single rib or a pressure sore on a bony prominence in a nutritionally-depleted patient. Regional distress is produced by processes, such as obstructive lymphedema, partial obstruction of a hollow viscus, or vascular compromise of an extremity. Generalized distress is typified by meningeal carcinomatosis that causes widespread neuropathic pain syndromes, biliary obstruction that causes jaundice and symptoms of liver failure, paraneoplastic syndromes, and anorexia/cachexia syndrome of the common bile duct with its consequence of severe metabolic impairment or complete bowel obstruction that leads to intractable nausea and vomiting with rapid dehydration.

Descriptive classification schemes for the selection of palliative treatment can be used as well. Examples include effusions; complications related to rapid, uncontrolled tumor growth; obstruction of a viscus; extensive infiltration of a secretory organ; acute or chronic bleeding; and uncontrolled pain.

What is feasible and what is possible

When the assessment of patient factors is complete, planning for a procedure should consider what is feasible and possible. Constraints should be identified and ideally should be discussed with an interdisciplinary team. The insights of the palliative care team members can identify issues that arise from the different domains in which they have professional expertise (eg, social work, spiritual care). The principles and preparation for a palliative procedure essentially are the same for any of the body areas. Appendix 1 details examples of palliative surgical procedures by body area or organ systems and general considerations in selection [4,8,12–15].

Many patients who require palliative surgical procedures also have significant anesthetic risks. Preoperative consults from an anesthesiologist often will avoid last minute cancellations, permit comprehensive planning of an anesthetic, and greatly improve perioperative care of these patients.

Rescinding "do not resuscitate" and "do not intubate" orders before any anesthetic for patients who have these advance directives is an ongoing problem in many institutions [16]. Informed consent also is an issue. The clear identification of the health care proxy for a patient and decision process that a family has in place should be resolved well before the surgical date.

Pain management is a consideration in any palliative surgical procedure, as part of the ongoing assessment of any patient who receives palliative care and for pain that is caused by the procedure itself. Patients who are on chronic opioid therapy can have a substantial increase or decrease in opioid requirements after any procedure, depending on the opioid-sparing effect of the procedure. Overdosage can occur, even in opioid-tolerant patients, if high dosages of opioids that previously were necessary for the relief of pain continue to be given after the pain is eliminated suddenly (eg, after a neuroablative procedure); however, overzealous tapering of opioids can precipitate an opioid withdrawal syndrome. Pain management expertise that was engaged preoperatively can be helpful for these patients, especially if neuraxial approaches (eg, epidural catheter placement) are to be considered. In some cases, these interventions can "double dip" by providing the anesthetic means and postprocedural pain control.

Spiritual and psychosocial factors

Religious and spiritual beliefs should be addressed in all care planning for patients and their families when considering palliative surgical care [17]. Treatment decisions often can be based on spiritual beliefs or religious preferences whether verbalized or not. When these concerns are raised, the patient's treating team should listen empathetically and attempt to gain insight into the core beliefs. Clergy, in addition to those who may be on the palliative care team, may be necessary to bring about an understanding of a family's belief system.

The importance of collegiality between the surgeon and those who are entrusted with spiritual care of the patient who is undergoing palliative surgery was emphasized 30 years ago [18]. The belief in miracles that many patients and families have in life-threatening diseases should not be confronted in any discussion, although care should be taken to avoid premature reassurance. The temptation to venture beyond one's own expertise about another's religious or spiritual beliefs should be resisted. Trying to resolve unanswerable questions quickly for a patient is likely to be a manifestation of the physician's own spiritual anxiety. Goals of these discussions should be clarification of concerns, establishment of a connection with the patient and the family, finding support for the patient, and determination of common goals of treatment and care as needed for clinical decisions.

In addition to general beliefs, specific religious or spiritual prohibitions or instructions regarding medical treatments should be identified. Examples of this include the proscription of blood transfusions for Jehovah's Witnesses and the care that is required by some beliefs for amputated body parts. This discussion also should address the belief system's attitude about the meaning and limits of medical support.

Psychologic considerations beyond the baseline assessment of cognitive and affective function include the potential psychologic impact of procedures, such as stoma formation, external catheter drainage, and prosthetics. For the insightful surgeon, witnessing the coping mechanisms of a patient/family who is anticipating some loss of control (undergoing general anesthesia and surgery) can give a clue about the nature of future adaptation during the process of dying.

Practical and economic concerns related to a planned procedure may be the most pressing issue for some patients. Few surgeons have the background that is necessary to provide direction on these matters; however, they never can go wrong by soliciting advice from social workers, therapists, and others who participate in follow-up care. The information from these members of the interdisciplinary team can influence consent. Complete care and appreciation of the impact on a patient's daily life should be discussed in detail before proceeding with any procedure. Even in situations where the care is required and few options exist, the time that is spent discussing what will be needed is appreciated greatly by the family and is fundamental in maintaining a positive therapeutic relationship with the family.

Health care resources

Few patients have unlimited resources for health care. Given the inaccuracy of life expectancy projections, financial considerations always are a significant consideration for patients. Procedures that require ongoing professional care are expensive and are not always covered completely by a patient's insurance plan. Treatment plans can vary based on financial resources alone.

Treatment considerations, therefore, should include the discharge plan [19]. The discharge planning process should begin early in the hospital course and should be based on the family's wishes and capacity to absorb the additional responsibilities that can occur. Most patients and families believe that the primary goal of most patients is to go home again and spend the last period of life there. Although this is ideal, a significant number of families do not have the resources, capacity, or wish to accomplish this. The key to understanding these barriers and making the correct decisions about potential palliative surgical approaches is an ongoing, open, honest, and frank discussion that is backed up by the full resources of an interdisciplinary team.

Perioperative management

Most patients who are considered for a palliative surgical procedure likely will have chronic pain that requires treatment with chronic opioid therapy. Patients who are on chronic opioid therapy are at a much higher risk of poorly-managed pain and cognitive impairment in the perioperative period. Guidelines for these patients are outlined in Table 2 [20–23]. In addition, these patients are at significant risk for perioperative delirium [24]. Repeated and careful assessment of each patient for evolving delirium can detect the prodromal signs of loss of orientation and decrease in cognitive ability that should prompt consideration of immediate treatment. Rapid recognition and treatment of delirium can prevent the full presentation of this disconcerting syndrome that can prolong hospital stay significantly, increase family distress, and lead to an increased risk of substantial complications [25].

Summary

Palliative surgical care should not be reserved for the end of a patient's life. The increasing emphasis on a patient's quality of life within the scope of

Table 2
Perioperative analgesic management in patients undergoing chronic opioid therapy

Action	Rationale
Determine total opioid dosage, often expressed as morphine equivalents.	Helpful for the needed dose conversions that will be required when switching from one opioid to another and for converting from oral to intravenous route.
Determine baseline mental status, address concerns about available analgesic approaches, and provide reassurance that the patient's concerns about pain management are addressed.	Neuroaxial and regional anesthetic techniques using catheters can be useful for effective pain management in patients who are opioid tolerant.
Maintain baseline opioids in the immediate preoperative period.	Prevent pain flares and unnecessary withdrawal. Be prepared to provide the equivalent dose IV if needed.
Patients will require substantial increases of opioids in both the intraoperative and postoperative periods. Use continuous opioid infusions with all patient-controlled analgesia regimens.	The increase in postoperative pain seen in patients who have chronic opioid therapy can last much longer than in patients who are not undergoing chronic opioid therapy.
If the operative procedure eliminates the source or perception of pain (eg, neurolytic procedure), postoperative opioid dosing will need to be substantially less than preoperative chronic dosage.	To prevent opioid withdrawal syndrome, taper previous day's 24-h dosage by 25% every few days until the daily dosage is 30 mg in morphine equivalents [43,44].
Use adjuvant analgesics and pre-emptive analgesic approaches.	Allows opioid sparing, which can decrease undesirable opioid-related side effects. Increases likelihood of postoperative pain control.

medical care and innovation within the field of surgery have made palliative surgery an increasingly desirable option for the control of distressing symptoms of an incurable disease, regardless of the impact on the disease process. Effective palliative surgery must widen its future perspective to acknowledge the impact of chronic illness upon the patient's family and support system and include this consideration in preoperative planning.

Because patients who have advanced disease typically can have multiple symptoms, careful assessment through active questioning of the patient and family offers the best chance to select treatment that can avoid redundancy. When planning and preparing a patient for palliative surgery, the focus of the procedure should be on resolving symptoms that are active and relevant to the patient but not at the expense of future quality of life.

Multidisciplinary teams are used often to provide palliative care because of the variety of needs that a patient and family may have. As a welcome, new member of the interdisciplinary team, the surgeon should rely on the information that the team has gathered in the planning of a palliative surgical procedure. Palliative procedures can be just as intellectually and emotionally gratifying to the surgeon as curative procedures with the added benefit that, when done well, they are appreciated deeply by patients and families because they know that the willingness to improve quality of life requires genuine interest.

Appendix 1. Classification of palliative procedure considerations by body region and selected systems

Head, eye, neck, and throat

Bleeding or threatened bleeding:

- **Epistaxis:** anterior and posterior nasal packing, balloon tamponade (30-cc Foley), silver nitrate cauterization, endoscopic cauterization, arterial embolization, ligation of internal maxillary artery ± anterior/posterior ethmoid arteries, ligation by way of maxillary sinus (Caldwell-Luc approach)
- **Operative or tumor site bleeding or threatened bleeding:** endoscopic cauterization; external carotid artery ligation; other vascular ligations; grafting of irradiated, ulcerated areas using myocutaneous (delto-pectoral) flaps

Blindness: intraocular instillation of antiviral agents for HIV-related infections of the retina, excision of cataracts due to radiation and other ocular therapies

Disfigurement and functional loss: debulking of tumor, autologous tissue grafting with or without prosthetics

Dysphagia: resection or debulking of tumor

Dysphonia (hoarseness): stenting of true vocal cords in instances of recurrent laryngeal nerve dysfunction

Dyspnea: resection of obstructing lesions of the tongue or pharynx or debulking using endoscopic electrocautery, cryosurgery, or laser. Subtotal thyroidectomy for bulky lesions of the thyroid with tracheal compression. Open or percutaneous tracheostomy for fixed upper airway obstruction, access for suctioning copious secretions, or reduced work of breathing in chronic ventilatory insufficiency.

Pain: resection or debulking as in treatment for dyspnea, nerve section, stellate ganglion block, dental extractions for painful caries or abscess, enucleation for painful, blind eye.

General considerations:

- The local impact of neoplastic disease is functionally and cosmetically far more disruptive than disease that arises elsewhere in the body. Most patients who have head and neck cancer die with local and regional disease only.

- Because of numerous specialized functions of the head and oral cavity (eg, facial expression, speech, chewing, swallowing), an interdisciplinary approach, including speech and other specialized therapists, is essential in planning surgical intervention.
- Consider adjuvant therapies, such as radiation therapy, because of the limited tissue that is available for resection and closure with its impact on cosmesis and function.
- Cryosurgery and laser resection can be used for debulking (cytoreduction) in previously irradiated fields where repeat radiation treatment is not normally feasible because of dose limitations.
- Some procedures may require the participation of neurologic, ophthalmologic, reconstructive, vascular, and abdominal surgeons.
- Many of the principles and techniques (debridement, resection, and autologous tissue cover) that are used in the management of surgical wounds or lesions of the head and neck can be applied to similar problems that occur in the breast or extremities.

Chest

Aspiration: Tracheoesphogeal fistula—endoscopic stenting with non-fenestrated stent [26], esophageal resection

Bleeding: endobronchial resection and cauterization, arterial embolization, lung resection

Dysphagia: esophageal stenting, endoluminal resection, photodynamic therapy, esophageal resection by way of thorocotomy or substernal approaches in carefully selected cases

Dyspnea: see article by Mentzer elsewhere in this issue

- *Pleural effusion:* thoracentesis, thoracostomy, thoraco-peritoneal shunt [27], talc pleurodesis (open and thoracoscopic), and decortication for pleural effusion
- *Parenchymal abnormalities:* bullectomy for localized emphysematous disease, marsupialization of emphysematous bulla, lung volume reduction surgery for diffuse emphysematous disease [28]
- *Ventilatory compromise:* decortication of trapped lung, thorocoplasty
- *Airway obstruction:* endobronchial resection using laser ablation, electrocautery, cryotherapy, radiation (brachytherapy), and photodynamic therapy [29], endobronchial stenting, tracheo-bronchial stenting by way of tracheostomy
- *Pericardial effusions:* percutaneous drainage under ultrasound guidance [30]; pericardial fenestration by subxyphoid, thorocotomy, or video-assisted thoracoscopic approaches; pericardioperitoneal shunting [31]; balloon pericardiotomy

- *Pericardial disease:* pericardiectomy for nonneoplastic constrictive pericarditis for relief of dyspnea and anasarca
- *Mediastinal disease:* superior vena cava balloon dilatation or stenting, rarely vascular bypass for superior vena caval obstruction

Disfigurement: resection of chest wall masses, debulking, chest wall reconstruction, breast reconstruction

Pain: rib resection, tumor debulking, neurectomy, ganglion block

- *Anginal pain procedures:* coronary angioplasty and stenting, intra-aortic balloon pump, minimally-invasive coronary bypass procedures, transmyocardial laser revascularization, cervical block

Additional considerations:

- Surgical pleurodesis using talc poudrage at thoracoscopy or thoracotomy for the management of pleural effusion has a higher success rate than thoracentesis and chemical pleurodesis (>90% versus 50%–60%) [32]. Increased use of video-assisted thoracoscopy is replacing the need for open thoracotomy for pleurodesis and other procedures for the lung and chest cavity.
- Resection of lung parenchyma rarely indicated for palliative purposes. Incomplete tumor debulking does not prolong life or provide effective palliation unless coupled with effective adjuvant chemotherapy or radiation therapy.
- Symptoms that are due to endoluminal disease are more likely to respond to endoscopic interventions, whereas extrinsic compression of airways that is due to neoplasm is managed better using radiation therapy. Bronchoscopic approaches can be used in instances of failed radiation therapy and radiation therapy in the form of brachytherapy can be introduced following endoluminal obliteration of tumor and stenting. Availability, cost, and operator experience with these approaches vary widely.
- Self-expanding metal stents that are used in vascular, gastrointestinal, biliary, and urinary systems are more comfortable, easier to insert, and safer than the more rigid plastic stents, although they cannot be removed once placed (migration has been reported).
- A thoracoscopic and laparoscopic approach to esophagectomy is technically feasible and safe for the treatment of benign and malignant esophageal disease. With a mean follow-up of 26 months, thoracoscopic and laparoscopic esophagectomy seems to be an oncologically-acceptable surgical approach for the treatment of esophageal cancer [33].
- The results from debulking of pericardial tumor and tumors that cause superior vena caval obstruction generally are dismal
- Coronary bypass originally was introduced and was accepted rapidly for palliation of angina pectoris due to coronary artery disease before

improved survival also was demonstrated. Less invasive antianginal surgical procedures may be considered if anginal symptoms do not yield to medical therapy or medical therapy has side effects that are unacceptable to the patient, even in cases of short life expectancy due to cardiac disease or noncardiac disease.

Abdomen and pelvis

Bleeding:

- *Endoluminal bleeding:* endoscopic electro or laser cauterization for localized sources of bleeding; alcohol injection of bleeding ulcers; open or laparoscopic suture ligation of bleeding ulcers; total or subtotal gastrectomy for bulky, bleeding lesions of the stomach; bowel resection for single or multiple sources (melanoma)
- *Variceal bleeding:* endoscopic sclerotherapy, balloon tamponade, transjugular intrahepatic portosystemic shunt (TIPS) for variceal hemorrhage
- *Pelvic bleeding:* arteriography and embolization, arterial ligation

Dyspnea, bloating, rapid satiety:

- *Ascites:* needle paracentesis, "pigtail" catheter insertion, Tenkhoff (peritoneal dialysis catheter) insertion for drainage, Denver or Levine peritoneo-venous shunt, peritoneal-vesicle shunt, TIPS for ascites due to Budd-Chiarri syndrome (hepatic vein thrombosis), intracaval metallic stent placement
- *Mass or organomegaly:* splenectomy for massive splenomegaly, tumor debulking (liver, omentum, bowel)

Fistula: wound care, excision of tract and bowel resection, diversion by proximally-placed ostomy, stenting with nonfenestrated stent, intubation of fistulous tract.

Intestinal obstruction: percutaneous drainage of obstructed viscus, stenting, endoluminal resection, open or laparoscopic intubation of viscus (gastrostomy, jejunostomy, cecostomy), open or laparoscopic resection with or without ostomy, open or laparoscopic bypass with or without ostomy

Jaundice: percutaneous and endoscopic stenting of common bile duct, endoscopic sphincterotomy, endoscopic laser recanalization, cholecystojejunostomy, cholodochojejunostomy, hepaticojejunostomy, hepaticogastrostomy, ampullectomy, pancreatic head resection (Whipple operation), rarely, for palliation [34]

Extremity edema: groin lymphadenectomy may improve or slow the progression of severe upper and lower extremity edema due to metastatic breast disease or melanoma in select cases. Intracaval stenting for massive lower extremity edema secondary to compression of the inferior vena cava by intrahepatic tumor.

Pain: celiac plexus block, metastatectomy, debulking, endoluminal resection or ablation, laparoscopic sympathectomy

General considerations:

- Certain symptoms that are associated with systemic disease or disease of the chest have abdominal etiologies. Anorexia may be due to obstructive jaundice or massive splenomegaly, whereas dyspnea may be due to tense ascites.
- There has been general consensus that gastric resection is preferable to bypass procedures for the relief of symptoms (obstruction, bleeding, pain) due to neoplasms [35].
- There is little prospective data that compare efficacy or patient satisfaction regarding choice of invasive procedures for ascites. Factors in selection include: life-expectancy, underlying etiology of ascites, presence of coagulopathy and infection, degree of loculation of ascites, characteristics of ascites (eg, turbid, bloody), nature of abdominal wall and previous intraperitoneal surgery, and patient acceptance of an externalized drain.
- Favorable candidates for operative management of malignant intestinal obstruction include: age younger than 65 years; normal nutritional status; absence of palpable abdominal masses; absence of ascites; well-defined radiographic locus of obstruction; absence of previously failed chemotherapy and no previous abdominal radiation therapy [36]; patient's wish for surgery; marked abdominal distention that suggests the absence of extensive, infiltrative disease [37]. Contraindications include recent demonstration of extensive intra-abdominal disease at laparotomy, poor general condition, patient refusal, and multiple sites of obstruction.
- Surgical bypass and endoscopic stenting are equally effective for the relief of symptoms that are caused by obstructive jaundice that is due to malignancy. Earlier complications are greater for surgical bypass, whereas late complications are more frequent in patients who are treated endoscopically. Surgical bypass may be more desirable in healthier patients who have longer life expectancy and is the preferred approach for patients who have coexisting duodenal obstruction.
- Consider placement of a vena cava filter as an adjunct to abdominal, pelvic, and orthopedic palliative procedures in hypercoagulable patients in whom mechanical or pharmacologic prophylaxis would be undesirable.

Genitourinary system

Hematuria: nephrectomy, bladder resection, tumor debulking, vessel ligation or embolization, cystoscopic coagulation, infusion of sclerosing agents by way of urinary catheter, arterial perfusion

Systemic symptoms (eg, fever, malaise, weight loss, anorexia): nephrectomy for renal cell carcinoma even in the presence of distant metastases [38], bladder resection for bulky lesions

Fistula: diversion; resection; stenting for fistulas to colon, vagina, and skin. Ureteric occlusion combined with percutaneous nephrostomy for perineal urinary fistula [39].

Outflow obstruction: ureteral catheter drainage, percutaneous suprapubic cystostomy, transurethral resection

Pain: ureteral stenting for pain due to hydronephrosis, kidney or bladder resection for tumor pain, penectomy for tumor-related pain and odor, transurethral resection or debulking of tumor causing pain, castration for hormonal manipulation of tumor in management of painful bony metastases as an alternative to pharmacotherapy

Uremic symptoms due to obstructive uropathy: ureteral stenting using antegrade, retrograde or combination approaches; percutaneous nephrostomy; hemodialysis as a temporizing measure until condition and goals can be clarified [40]

Impotence: implantable prosthesis

- For initial management of gross hematuria, insert a larger bore urinary catheter (20–24 French) with triple ports to allow for irrigation as well as drainage.
- Ultrasonography is the procedure of choice for confirmation of hydronephrosis because pyelography dye is contraindicated or may not visualize in these patients.
- Retrograde, antegrade, and combination approaches can be used for ureteral stenting. The retrograde approach is preferred but is not always possible because of tumor distortion of the bladder trigone. Subcutaneously-placed urinary stents have been described [41]. Percutaneous nephrostomy for relief of malignant obstruction was associated with less prohibitive mortality and morbidity than open procedures [42].

Skeletal system

Pain with impending fracture or established pathological fracture:

- *Weight bearing:* operative reduction/radiation therapy, nonoperative immobilization and analgesics, blocks
- *Non–weight-bearing:* radiation therapy, nonoperative immobilization and analgesics, blocks
- *Vertebral:* analgesics, blocks, vertebroplasty (kyphoplasty)

Spinal instability or collapse: operative fixation

Cord compression: operative decompression, steroids, radiation therapy, chemotherapy

- See article by Aboulafia and Sagini elsewhere in this issue for further discussion of orthopedic management.
- Symptom control for skeletal system symptoms from benign and malignant disease usually requires pharmacotherapy and physical therapy as parts of a chronic, comprehensive management program (eg, analgesics, bisphosphonates hormonal therapy/replacement, massage).

Nervous system

Peripheral nerves: lysis, debulking, neurectomy
Autonomic nervous system: splanchnicectomy (chemical, using alcohol)
Spinal cord: decompression and stabilization
Brain: see article by Barker elsewhere in this issue

- Infiltration can cause various pain syndromes. Surgical resection can have significant side effects. Avoid resection whenever possible. In cases of tumor infiltration of nerve, surgical resection rarely is helpful.
- Surgical decompression often is emergent if weakness is progressive and radiation is not effective
- Para- or quadriplegia is has a detrimental effect on quality of life and complicates the patient's care considerably

References

[1] Bruera E, Neumann CM. Management of specific symptom complexes in patients receiving palliative care. CMAJ 1998;158(13):1717–26.
[2] Quill TE, Dresser R, Brock DW. The rule of double effect—a critique of its role in end-of-life decision making. N Engl J Med 1997;337(24):1768–71.
[3] Billings JA. Recent advances: palliative care. BMJ 2000;321(7260):555–8.
[4] Ripamonti C, Twycross R, Baines M, et al. Clinical-practice recommendations for the management of bowel obstruction in patients with end-stage cancer. Support Care Cancer 2001;9(4):223–33.
[5] Carver AC, Foley KM. Symptom assessment and management. Neurol Clin 2001;19(4): 921–47.
[6] Galer BS, Henderson J, Perander J, et al. Course of symptoms and quality of life measurement in Complex Regional Pain Syndrome: a pilot survey. J Pain Symptom Manage 2000;20(4):286–92.
[7] Hume M. Improving care at the end of life. Qual Lett Healthc Lead 1998;10(10):2–10.
[8] Levy MH, Rosen SM, Ottery FD, et al. Supportive care in oncology. Curr Probl Cancer 1992;16(6):329–418.
[9] Faulkner A. ABC of palliative care. Communication with patients, families, and other professionals. BMJ 1998;316(7125):130–2.
[10] Watanabe S, Bruera E. Anorexia and cachexia, asthenia, and lethargy. Hematol Oncol Clin North Am 1996;10(1):189–206.
[11] Sutton LM, Demark-Wahnefried W, Clipp EC. Management of terminal cancer in elderly patients. Lancet Oncol 2003;4(3):149–57.

[12] Meyerson BA. Neurosurgical approaches to pain treatment. Acta Anaesthesiol Scand 2001;
     45(9):1108–13.
[13] Hunstad DA, Norton JA. Management of pancreatic carcinoma. Surg Oncol 1995;4(2):
     61–74.
[14] Ashburn MA, Lipman AG. Management of pain in the cancer patient. Anesth Analg 1993;
     76(2):402–16.
[15] Dunn G, Johnson A, editors. Surgical palliative care, vol. 1. 1st edition. New York: Oxford
     University Press; 2004.
[16] Anesthesiologists. Ethical guidelines for the anesthesia care of patients with do-not-
     resuscitate orders or other directives that limit treatment. 2001. Available at: http://
     www.asahg.org/publicationsAndServices/standards/09.html.
[17] Lo B, Ruston D, Kates LW, et al. Discussing religious and spiritual issues at the end of life:
     a practical guide for physicians. JAMA 2002;287(6):749–54.
[18] Gaisford JC. Palliative surgery. JAMA 1972;221:81–4.
[19] Emanuel EJ, Fairclough DL, Slutsman J, et al. Assistance from family members, friends,
     paid care givers, and volunteers in the care of terminally ill patients. N Engl J Med 1999;
     341(13):956–63.
[20] Warltier D, Mitra S, Sinatra R. Perioperative management of acute pain in the opioid-
     dependant patient. Anesthesiology 2004;101(1):1–28.
[21] Goldstein FJ. Adjuncts to opioid therapy. J Am Osteopath Assoc 2002;102(9 Suppl 3):
     S15–21.
[22] Osenbach RK, Harvey S. Neuraxial infusion in patients with chronic intractable cancer and
     noncancer pain. Curr Pain Headache Rep 2001;5(3):241–9.
[23] Sandler AN. Post-thoracotomy analgesia and perioperative outcome. Minerva Anestesiol
     1999;65(5):267–74.
[24] Casarett DJ, Inouye SK. Diagnosis and management of delirium near the end of life. Ann
     Intern Med 2001;135(1):32–40.
[25] Ross DD, Alexander CS. Management of common symptoms in terminally ill patients: Part
     II. Constipation, delirium and dyspnea. Am Fam Physician 2001;64(6):1019–26.
[26] Do YS, Song HY, Lee BH, et al. Esophagorespiratory fistula associated with esophageal
     cancer: treatment with a Gianturco stent tube. Radiology 1993;187:673–7.
[27] Petrou M, Kaplan D, Goldstraw P. Management of recurrent malignant pleural effusions.
     The complementary role talc pleurodesis and pleuroperitoneal shunting. Cancer 1995;75(3):
     801–5.
[28] Cooper JD, Patterson GA. Lung-volume reduction surgery for severe emphysema. Chest
     Surg Clin North Am 1995;5(4):815–31.
[29] Baas P, van Zandwijk N. Endobronchial treatment modalities in thoracic oncology. Ann
     Oncol 1995;6(6):523–31.
[30] Tsang TS, Seward JB, Barnes ME, et al. Outcomes of primary and secondary treatment of
     pericardial effusion in patients with malignancy. Mayo Clinic Proc 2000;75:248–53.
[31] Fiocco M, Krasna MJ. The management of malignant pleural and pericardial effusions.
     Hematol Oncol Clin North Am 1997;11:253–65.
[32] Hartman DL, Gaither JM, Kesler KA, et al. Comparison of insufflated talc under
     thoracoscopic guidance with standard tetracycline and bleomycin pleurodesis for control of
     malignant pleural effusions [randomized controlled trial]. J Thor Cardiovasc Surg 1993;
     105(4):743–7 [discussion 747–8].
[33] Nguyen NT, Roberts P, Follette DM, et al. Thoracoscopic and laparoscopic esophagectomy
     for benign and malignant disease: lessons learned from 46 consecutive procedures. J Am Coll
     Surg 2003;197(6):902–13.
[34] Lillemoe KD, Cameron JL, Yeo CJ, et al. Pancreaticodudenectomy. Does it have a role in
     the palliation of pancreatic cancer? Ann Surg 1996;223:718–28.
[35] Doglietto GB, Pacelli F, Caprino P, et al. Palliative surgery for far-advanced gastric cancer:
     a retrospective study on 305 consecutive patients. Am J Surg 1999;65:352–5.

[36] Krebs H, Gobelrud DR. Surgical management of bowel obstruction in advanced ovarian carcinoma. Obstet Gynecol 1983;61:327–30.

[37] Baines MJ. The medical management of malignant intestinal obstruction. Baillieres Clin Oncol 1987;1:357–71.

[38] Couillard DR, deVere White RW. Surgery of renal cell carcinoma. Urol Clin North Am 1993;20(2):263–75.

[39] Barton DP, Morse SS, Fiorica JV, et al. Percutaneous nephrostomy and ureteral stenting in gynecologic malignancies. Obstet Gynecol 1992;85:805–11.

[40] Fainsinger RL. Integrating medical and surgical treatments in gastrointestinal, genitourinary, and biliary obstruction in patients with cancer. Hematol Oncol Clin North Am 1996; 10(1):173–88.

[41] Ahmadzadeh M. Clinical experience with subcutaneous urinary diversion: new approach using a double pigtail stent. Br J Urol 1991;67(6):596–9.

[42] Culkin DJ, Wheeler JS Jr, Marsans RE, et al. Percutaneous nephrostomy for palliation of metastatic ureteral obstruction. Urology 1987;30(3):229–31.

[43] Hanks G, Cherny N, Fallon M. Opioid analgesic therapy. In: Doyle D, Hanks G, Cherny N, et al, editors. Oxford textbook of palliative medicine. 3rd edition. Philadelphia: Oxford University Press; 2003. p. 316–41.

[44] Management of cancer pain. Clinical Practice Guideline No. 9. US Department of Health and Human Services; 1994. AHCPR Publication No. 94–0592.

ELSEVIER
SAUNDERS

SURGICAL
CLINICS OF
NORTH AMERICA

Surg Clin N Am 85 (2005) 209–224

Chronic Pain Management in the Surgical Patient

A. Reed Thompson, MD, FACS[a,*], Jonathan J. Wolfe, PhD, RPh[b]

[a]*Donald W. Reynolds Department of Geriatrics, University of Arkansas for Medical Sciences, 4301 West Markham Street, Slot 748, Little Rock, AR 72205, USA*
[b]*Department of Pharmacy Practice, College of Pharmacy, University of Arkansas for Medical Sciences, 4301 W. Markham Street, Slot 522, Little Rock, AR 72205, USA*

Surgeons are accustomed to treating pain. Surgery plays an integral part in the management of many painful conditions, and treating pain through the perioperative period is a core competency of surgeons; however, managing patients who have chronic pain has not been a high priority in surgical practice. Although a significant number of surgical patients have chronic pain, its management generally has been delegated to others in the health care system. The education of surgeons in the management of chronic pain has been minimal to date. Modern textbooks of surgery discuss the management of chronic pain only briefly.

Although surgery does not have a central role in the management of chronic pain, surgeons could have a role in its management. Pain may persist after curative or palliative surgical procedures, and patients often look to their surgeon for help when it does. Armed with some basic knowledge and skills, surgeons could feel more comfortable in continuing to care for their patients who are in chronic pain and strengthening the bond between patient and surgeon as discussed by Lee et al [1].

This article provides some basic information on the management of chronic pain that may improve surgeons' participation in the care of their patients whose pain persists after surgical procedures have been completed. Although the primary intervention for chronic pain is drug therapy, its optimal management requires a multi-disciplinary approach. Nonpharmacologic and pharmacologic interventions for chronic pain in the surgical patient are discussed.

---

* Corresponding author.
E-mail address: arthompson@uams.edu (A.R. Thompson).

0039-6109/05/$ - see front matter © 2005 Elsevier Inc. All rights reserved.
doi:10.1016/j.suc.2004.12.003   *surgical.theclinics.com*

Definition of chronic pain

Chronic or persistent pain can be defined as pain that lasts for more than 3 to 6 months. Pain that last for weeks beyond the expected time that is required for healing to occur after an injury; pain that is associated with a persistent active pathologic process; and episodic pain that recurs over months also can be defined as chronic [2]. Chronic pain commonly is divided into malignant and nonmalignant categories because there are some differences in the approach to management. Pain from a nonmalignant source is likely to have a longer course; more often requires the use of multidimensional pain assessment tools, such as the Brief Pain Inventory [3]; and benefits from multiple modalities of therapy in its management than does pain from a malignant source. Providers often also display an attitudinal difference: if the pain cannot be "seen" (eg, vague abdominal pain after an exploratory laparotomy versus pain from a bone metastasis in breast cancer that can be "seen" on a bone scan), it is less likely to be addressed optimally. Nonetheless, the basic principles in management apply to malignant and nonmalignant pain.

Barriers to optimal chronic pain management in the surgical patient

Managing patients' chronic pain has not been a priority in surgical care or in the education of surgeons (Box 1). If the same comprehensive attitude toward the management of chronic pain existed in surgical training that has existed for decades in the management of postoperative

---

Box 1. Barriers to optimal chronic pain management in surgical patients

Surgeons
Low priority
Knowledge deficits in pain assessment and pharmacology
   of analgesic agents

Patients
Failure to report pain
Concerns about addiction

Health care system
Low priority
Lack of practice standards
Regulatory environment

wound complications, surgeons would be the nation's experts in the management of chronic pain. Because surgeons already deal on a daily basis with patients who are in pain, the learning curve for improving the management of chronic pain promises to be short and steep. It would only require a small addition to the curriculum of surgical training programs and minor additions to the continuing education programs of practicing surgeons. Improvement in the management of the surgical patient who is in chronic pain is only a matter of reprioritizing chronic pain to a more important position in surgical care.

Information on technologies for managing chronic pain has been available for years. It is the poor dissemination of knowledge to providers that acts as a barrier to chronic pain management. Two of the most common areas of knowledge deficit are in pain assessment and opioid analgesic use. Both can be overcome easily and are discussed here.

Some patient-centered barriers also demand solutions. Patients, particularly older patients, regularly underreport their pain. This phenomenon seems to be related to several factors. Our culture often communicates a bias against reporting pain, because that can be interpreted as a sign of weakness. Many older patients underreport their pain because they believe that pain is a normal part of aging; actually, the presence of pain always means pathology. Patient denial can reduce pain complaints. To patients who have a serious illness (eg, cancer), pain means that their disease may be active, and denial is a defense mechanism. Patients also may choose to suffer with their pain unnecessarily, rather than to complain because they fear that mentioning the pain may lead to more painful procedures. Patients often do not want to take opioid drugs because of concerns about loss of cognition and functional status and fear of addiction. This prejudice persists despite the reality that compounds in the opioid drug family are the appropriate mainstay for chronic pain management for many patients. Information on the dangers of opioid analgesics is replete in our society, but information on their benefits and that legitimate medical indications exist for their use receives far less emphasis.

Our health care system produces barriers. There is a lack of system-wide standards in the management of chronic pain, although organizations, such as the American Geriatrics Society and the American Medical Directors Association, have published guidelines on its management [4,5]. There are no uniform practice standards proposed by surgeons for chronic pain management in the surgical patient.

The drug regulatory atmosphere in our health care system acts as a barrier. The regulatory environment at the state and federal levels was shown to act as a deterrent in the prescribing and dispensing of opioid analgesics, which are the mainstay in the management of moderate and severe chronic pain [6]. Knowledge of one's current local regulatory board position on the prescribing of controlled substances for chronic pain is essential in today's practice environment.

A brief look at pain physiology

Pain processes are complex, particularly in central processing where a neural stimulus becomes a pain experience. Despite the complexity of these neural processes, two distinct pain mechanisms—nociceptive and neuro-pathic—can be identified. This has important clinical relevance because the response to treatment of the two mechanisms differs [7]. The nociceptive pain mechanism—subdivided into somatic and visceral types—is the mechanism that relays a pain signal through ascending pathways beginning with peripheral nerve fibers, to the dorsal root ganglion, decussating in the dorsal horn of the spinal column, then ascending the spinothalamic tracts to the thalamus, and on to cortical centers. The relay of neural signals along this pathway is an important natural process that can be considered essential to an organism's safety, preservation of function, and overall well-being. The nociceptive pain experience is protective, and therefore, has "meaning." Conversely, the neuropathic pain mechanism is considered to be an aberrant process. Stimuli that produce neuropathic pain originate from damaged neurons, and exercise no protective component for the organism. Neuro-pathic pain has no "meaning." The pain experience can be a mix of these two mechanisms, or it can arise through an unidentifiable, or idiopathic, process.

Identification of mechanisms in chronic pain is more complex than in acute pain. Chronic pain often is multi-factorial. Coexisting psychophysi-ologic conditions complicate the pain experience, and thus, the report of pain. Even so, identification of the pain mechanism typically can be done through comprehensive pain assessment.

Chronic pain assessment

The management of chronic pain in the surgical patient begins with a comprehensive pain assessment. The goals of pain assessment are to determine the severity of the pain and the basic pain mechanism that is responsible for it; this ultimately should lead to a pain diagnosis. Only then can appropriate pain treatment be implemented.

Chronic pain problems are distinctly different in presentation from the acute pain problems that surgeons are more accustomed to managing. Important differences in the presenting characteristics of acute and chronic pain contribute to the difficulty in assessing chronic pain (Table 1) [8]. Patients who are in chronic pain often have an ill-defined onset of their pain; they display no pain behaviors (moaning, splinting, wincing) even when pain is reported as severe; they have no autonomic signs (tachycardia, sweating, hypertension); and their pain often is associated with depression. A much more thorough assessment frequently is required to determine the pain mechanism and to arrive at a pain diagnosis in patients who have chronic pain.

Table 1
Acute and chronic pain differences

	Acute	Chronic
Temporal	Specific, well-defined onset	Vague, ill-defined onset
Intensity	Variable	Variable
Associated affect	Anxious	Irritable, depressed
Pain behavior	Moaning, splinting, rocking	May give no external indications
Autonomic signs	Diaphoresis, tachycardia	None
Meaning of pain	Warning	None

Adapted from Portenoy RK, Kanner RM, editors. Pain management: theory and practice. Philadelphia: FA Davis; 2003. p. 7.

All pain—acute and chronic, malignant and nonmalignant—is a subjective experience. Patient reports of pain should be believed until there is strong reason for doubt. Psychologic factors, such as anxiety and depression, influence the chronic pain experience. Their careful assessment is an essential part of chronic pain management [9]. The emotional and psychologic aspects of chronic pain often need to be assessed by mental health specialists.

Assessment begins with a history and a physical examination. A thorough history of past and present illnesses is supplemented by a pain history, which includes obtaining information about the pain quality, location, intensity, response to previous interventions, and current drug therapy, including alternative and complementary drugs.

Determining the pain quality helps to distinguish between the nociceptive and neuropathic pain mechanisms; this is important because pain from these two distinct mechanisms responds differently to analgesics. Nociceptive pain can be somatic or visceral in origin. When it is somatic, it has an aching, throbbing, occasionally sharp quality and the source of the pain usually is point-specific. Visceral pain has the same descriptors as somatic pain, but it frequently also has a cramping component. Visceral pain usually is reported as having a vague, rather than specific, location. Neuropathic pain is reported as a burning, hot, tingling, "on fire" sensation. It can be described as pain that radiates along a nerve root; sometimes a lancinating quality is described (Box 2). Pain also can be mixed—nociceptive/neuropathic—in origin.

Various validated pain assessment scales are available to assist in the measurement of pain intensity [10,11]. Assigning a pain score from 0 to 10 is a simple, straightforward clinical method of measuring pain intensity. Pain scores are particularly useful in monitoring patients who have chronic pain over time. The history should include inquiries on the effects of pain on activities of daily living, mood, and sleep. History of comorbid medical conditions, mental illness, and a history of substance abuse is important to assess.

The physical examination includes a careful examination of the painful site for signs of tenderness and inflammation. The neurologic examination

---

Box 2. Pain mechanisms and pain quality

Nociceptive
Somatic: aching, throbbing, sharp; well-defined location
Visceral: aching, throbbing, sharp, frequently cramping;
    vague location

Neuropathic
Hot, burning, tingling, "on fire"
Occasionally radiating or lancinating

---

includes evaluation of sensory, motor, and autonomic changes in the affected area. Radiographic studies frequently are indicated before a pain diagnosis can be made. Laboratory assessment of liver and renal function may be necessary, particularly when drug therapies are planned. The latter are especially important for treatment planning in older patients. Review of the history, physical examination, and all radiographic and laboratory findings usually leads to a pain diagnosis after which a plan of care can be developed.

Chronic pain treatment

The goal of chronic pain treatment is to improve the patient's quality of life by relieving pain and improving functional status. After a pain diagnosis has been established and the pain mechanism determined, a pain treatment plan should be developed and discussed with the patient. Patient education as to realistic goals of treatment was shown to improve outcomes in chronic pain management and it is an important part of the treatment plan [12]. Compliance with treatment recommendations is greater when the patient becomes a partner in long-term treatment. Compliance is facilitated further by continued physician–patient communication over time.

Because of the physiologic and psychologic complexities of chronic pain, multiple modalities of treatment frequently are necessary to approach success. Drug therapy is the mainstay in the treatment of chronic pain; but because pharmacologic and nonpharmacologic interventions can contribute to successful treatment, it is useful to know something about both approaches to therapy.

Nonpharmacologic interventions for chronic pain

Nonpharmacologic interventions for chronic pain generally supplement pharmacologic interventions (Box 3). They can be categorized as non-

---

Box 3. Nonpharmacologic interventions for chronic pain

Noninvasive
Behavioral and cognitive
   Relaxation
   Distraction
   Meditation
   Reframing
   Biofeedback
   Guided imagery

Physical and rehabilitative
Exercise
Cutaneous stimulation
   Superficial heat
   Superficial cold
   Massage
   Transcutaneous electrical nerve stimulation

Invasive
Anesthesia techniques
   Neural blockade
   Intraspinal drug infusions
Neurosurgical techniques
   Rhizotomy
   Cordotomy

Alternative and complimentary
Acupuncture
Manipulative/chiropractic methods

---

invasive and invasive. Noninvasive therapies include behavioral/cognitive therapies and physical/rehabilitative therapies. Invasive therapies range from trigger point injections through nerve ablation procedures to implantation of pumps and other devices.

Behavioral and cognitive therapies include such interventions as relaxation, distraction, meditation, reframing, guided imagery, and biofeedback [13]. Some are simple and easily learned, whereas others require a highly motivated patient. These are implemented best by referral to specialists in this area.

Physical and rehabilitative therapies include graded exercise programs and cutaneous stimulation techniques (eg, superficial heat and cold, massage) and neurostimulatory approaches (eg, transcutaneous electrical stimulation or percutaneous electrical stimulation). Specialists in this area can make major contributions toward achieving the therapeutic goals of pain relief and improved functional status. Consultation with them is encouraged in the management of difficult patients.

Invasive interventions can be useful in patients who have chronic pain; however, a small proportion of patients who have chronic pain require them. They include anesthesia and neurosurgical techniques. Anesthesia interventions include neural blocks, epidural steroid injections, and intraspinal administration of analgesics. Surgical interventions, such as rhizotomy and cordotomy, have made important contributions in the management of chronic pain in the past, but they rarely are indicated now. A discussion of them was published by Manchikanti et al [14].

Many patients who have chronic pain turn to alternative and complementary therapies. Most common are acupuncture and manipulative methods by chiropractic physicians. Anecdotal evidence suggests that acupuncture can have analgesic effects, but the mechanism remains unknown [15]. A meta-analysis of the published results of randomized, controlled clinical trials that evaluated acute and chronic back pain found that spinal manipulation was better than sham therapies, although not superior to conventional therapies [16].

Pharmacologic interventions for chronic pain

Pharmacologic interventions to control chronic pain will be judged by the effect that each patient experiences. The path to satisfactory pain control is staked out by the characteristics of the drugs themselves and the patient's response to them. Each drug has a unique pharmacology, pharmacodynamics, and pharmacokinetics. These separate elements combine with the characteristics of the particular patient to produce desirable therapeutic effects and undesirable side effects. Good and adverse effects are, to some degree, predictable; however, the drug regimen must be individualized in each patient for optimal outcome. Care to balance the beneficial and adverse effects of drug administration is essential in the treatment of chronic pain because therapy commonly persists for months or even years.

The pharmacology of analgesic drugs generally is well-established. Pharmacology concerns itself with the effects (beneficial and adverse) that can be associated reasonably with the chemical structure of a medication, including active ingredients and excipient chemicals that are used to produce a practical dosage form. Pharmacology tells a great deal about a drug, but it is incomplete without consideration of the other two domains, pharmacodynamics and pharmacokinetics. Pharmacodynamics concerns itself with the effect that is produced by a drug after it reaches the intended receptor. It is the key to gauging the appropriate dose for an expected effect. Pharmacokinetics studies the processes by which a particular drug is taken up by the body, transformed chemically by physiologic systems, and finally eliminated from the body.

Drug effects, in this case long-term efficacy in pain relief, and side effects arise from the interplay of all three elements of drug activity. It is not enough to select a product based on its pharmacology. The other two dimensions of the intended drug will go far toward making it practical and appropriate for a patient, or the basis for a therapeutic misadventure. The ideal drug for chronic pain will produce analgesia at a safe dose level and produce no side effects. The ideal drug will, moreover, have no target organ, in which it will produce a predictable, characteristic adverse effect.

Chronic nociceptive pain responds, to some degree, to virtually all conventional analgesic agents. Neuropathic pain, conversely, does not respond as well to any of the conventional agents, including most opioids. Optimal control of neuropathic pain usually requires the use of adjuvant analgesics.

Classes of drugs for treatment of chronic pain

Nonopioid analgesics

Nonsteroidal anti-inflammatory drugs

Nonsteroidal anti-inflammatory drugs (NSAIDs) constitute the class of drugs that is used most commonly and appropriately as mainstays in the treatment of chronic pain (Box 4). There are two basic types of NSAIDs, cyclo-oxygenase (COX) I inhibitors and COX II inhibitors; the latter have been available only in the last few years. The initial experience with COX II inhibitors demonstrated them to be better tolerated than COX I inhibitors; however; more recent experience challenges that information [17]. In September 2004, Merck and Co., Inc., (West Point, Pennsylvania) the manufacturers of Vioxx (rofecoxib), a COX-2 inhibitor, voluntarily withdrew this agent from the market over concerns of an increased risk of cardiovascular events (including heart attack and stroke). A comprehensive review of NSAID pharmacology has been published by the American Pain Society [18].

Their use is rational because inflammation commonly is a causal component of all pain. Chronic pain that is related to chronic pathologic processes (eg, arthritis, bony metastases) is likely to respond to anti-inflammatory drugs. The pharmacology of this class of agents predicts that their blockade of the arachidonic acid cascade will decrease the release of pain-causing agents into tissues that are impacted by the pathologic process. The World Health Organization analgesic ladder bases pain treatment on the use of NSAIDs.

NSAIDs are associated with a variety of problems from patient noncompliance with drug regimens to life-threatening hemorrhage. The predictable problem with NSAIDs is their adverse effect on the gastrointestinal (GI) tract. The GI effects of NSAIDs are well-known. Use of these drugs can produce irritation in the stomach that can progress to acute ulceration and bleeding, particularly in elderly patients. Nausea and

---

Box 4. Pharmacologic interventions for chronic pain

Nonopioid analgesics
Nonsteroidal anti-inflammatory drugs
Acetaminophen
Tramadol
Adjuvants
   Anticonvulsants
   Antidepressants

Opioid analgesics
Oral
  Immediate release
   Tablet
   Solution
  Extended release
  Rectal
  Transdermal
  Parenteral
   Intravenous
   Subcutaneous
   Intraspinal

---

vomiting can occur commonly with NSAID therapy in all ages. Renal toxicity from NSAIDs constitutes a particular concern. Because chronic pain frequently results from degenerative diseases that are related to aging and because creatinine clearance decreases with age, the kidneys are at a greater risk for toxicity in older patients. Thus, older patients require greater care in selection and monitoring of NSAIDs. NSAIDs also exhibit characteristic effects on the clotting cascade which requires great care to avoid drug-drug interactions. A good basic rule is to dose a basal NSAID up to the point of patient tolerance, and to continue that dosage unless a side effect appears. In most cases, the older patient will not tolerate a NSAID dosage that is nearly as high as the average healthy younger person. If one NSAID is not tolerated, it is possible that another one would be and could be tried before jettisoning the drug family completely.

The classic NSAID is aspirin. Its side effect profile is well-characterized. Like many NSAIDs, it is available over-the-counter (OTC). This fact makes aspirin and NSAIDs whose U.S. patents have expired more affordable than many other drugs. Although aspirin is the classic, it is not necessarily the drug to use first in the patient who has chronic pain. The choice should be that NSAID whose side effect profile best matches the needs of the patient.

The NSAIDs also are overlooked frequently in the pharmacologic management of chronic pain. Aspirin, ibuprofen, and acetaminophen are used as single agents. They also are combined with weak opioid drugs, such as codeine, in many analgesic products. The NSAID or acetaminophen content in the combination product limits the number of dosages, and therefore, the amount of opioid that a patient may receive. The result may be a subtherapeutic dosage and undertreated pain. A patient who receives an NSAID/opioid combination drug also can be placed at considerable risk by the use of OTC NSAIDs of which the prescriber and pharmacist are unaware.

For this reason alone it is necessary to take and to maintain an accurate drug history of any patient who is treated for chronic pain. Drugs that are approved by the U.S. Food and Drug Administration for sale OTC are approved only for specific maximum dosages and only for a limited time of use. Administration at higher than labeled doses or for longer than specified times, places patients at hazard. The hazard can arise from an underlying disease whose diagnosis is delayed by attempts at self-management, or from accumulation of a toxic dosage from overuse. Patients commonly do not appreciate the hazard from inappropriate use of OTC drugs; they believe them to safe because they may be bought without a prescription.

Acetaminophen. Generally, acetaminophen is well-tolerated and is a useful analgesic in the management of chronic pain. It commonly is considered in the same light as aspirin; however, acetaminophen has no anti-inflammatory effect, but rather is a centrally-acting analgesic and an antipyretic in its own right. Acetaminophen has the virtue of not affecting the clotting process, but it can interfere with the metabolism of warfarin and cause overanticoagulation [19]. Most experts believe that patients should not take more than 4000 mg/d because of its hepatic toxicity (acute and chronic). Patients have unlimited access to acetaminophen, and their total daily milligram consumption of OTC plus prescribed drug should be monitored carefully.

Tramadol

Tramadol is a weak μ-opioid agonist with low abuse potential. It has a dual mechanism of action, but it is not understood completely. Tramadol binds opioid receptors, and it inhibits the reuptake of norepinephrine and serotonin at nerve terminals. Its side effects are not fully reversible with the opioid antagonist, naloxone, and problems with dependence and addiction are unusual. Its use in patients who have chronic pain seems to be efficacious. It was reported to decrease the seizure threshold and should be used with caution in patients who have seizure disorders or those who receive other medications that also affect the seizure threshold.

Adjuvant analgesics

Adjuvant analgesics are used in the management of neuropathic pain. Meta-analysis of agents for neuropathic pain shows tricyclic antidepressants, anticonvulsants (gabapentin), local anesthetics (lidocaine patch), tramadol, and opioids are effective [20]. Drug dosages should be begun small and increased slowly to achieve optimal relief; however, the presence of neuropathic pain carries a guarded prognosis for relief, even with multiple-modality therapy.

Opioids

Opioid drugs are naturally occurring, synthetic, and semisynthetic compounds with profound analgesic properties. They stand next after NSAIDs for the management of chronic pain. Their use brings predictable hazards, but these commonly are overestimated in practice. The benefits of their use in chronic pain outweigh the burdens in many cases. Failure to appreciate fully the safety of opioids when appropriately prescribed for chronic pain is one of the barriers that is faced by many surgeons that can lead to undertreatment of pain. Three opioid pharmacologic properties contribute to their safety: lack of known organ toxicity, no ceiling, and tolerance.

Opioid drugs have the common virtue of having no known organ toxicity. Their primary effect is on μ and κ opioid receptors in the central and peripheral nervous systems, including sites in the spinal cord. The primary adverse effect of opioids is in the central nervous system, where overdosing can cause respiratory depression, somnolence, lethargy, and confusion. All of these effects are reversible with dose reductions and by administering an opioid antagonist (naloxone). The other main adverse effect is in the GI tract, where endogenous opioid receptors predictably produce constipation throughout the duration of opioid administration. Constipation can be managed readily and should not constitute a barrier to appropriate opioid therapy. Metabolites of particular opioids (eg, morphine-3-glucuronide) may present problems in particular patients with prolonged use, but these effects are reversible as the metabolite is cleared. The ability to rotate the pure opioid agonist drugs typically allows altering a patient's therapy to a tolerable analgesic without having to discontinue the entire drug class.

Opioid drugs also have no specific ceiling doses. There is no flattening of the opioid dose-response curve. Every dose increase in a patient who is habituated to pure opioid administration results in increased analgesia. Dose limitations are related to the presence of refractory side effects, rather than to a specific number of milligrams.

Tolerance is the other important aspect of opioid safety. It is defined as the need for increasing the drug dosage to achieve the same therapeutic effect. It is well-known that tolerance develops to the analgesic effect of opioids after prolonged use. Less well-known is that tolerance also develops to the opioid side effects. The linkage between opioid administration and respiratory depression is well-known. This is primarily an effect that is seen in opioid-naive patients. Respiratory depression typically diminishes with chronic opioid dosing as tolerance develops [21]. Respiratory depression may be associated with dosage increases in tolerant patients, but it is likely to be transitory and disappears as the central nervous system acclimates to the new higher dosage. In extreme cases, naloxone may be used to manage acute episodes of respiratory depression that impair dosage increases.

It is axiomatic that patients who receive chronic opioids will become dependent on the drug class; however, drug addiction usually does not occur. This drug dependence is defined as exhibition of withdrawal symptoms if the drug is discontinued abruptly. Drug addiction can be defined as impaired control over drug use, compulsive use and craving, and continued use despite harm. Drug dependence is not the same as drug addiction. Drug dependence is physiologic, whereas drug addiction is behavioral [7].

The management of chronic pain with opioid analgesics requires a simple and straightforward approach. The oral route of administration always is preferred. Patients are given a scheduled extended-release preparation around the clock and a supplemental immediate release preparation as needed for spikes in their pain. The opioid dosages are titrated to effect. The only limitation to the titration is the development of uncontrollable side effects, which requires dosage reduction or rotation to a different opioid. A laxative regimen always is added, except in circumstances of chronic diarrhea. The patients are followed regularly and their dosages are adjusted as indicated by the response to treatment. Long-term opioid use for pain relief seems to be safe, but there are potential adverse consequences with chronic opioid ingestion [22].

Best practice

The best practice in chronic pain management of surgical patients requires a comprehensive assessment and a multi-disciplinary treatment approach that uses nonpharmacologic and pharmacologic interventions. The patients need to have their treatment plan discussed clearly with them, and the plan should be documented in the medical record as an informed consent. The patients need to be seen on a regular basis for re-evaluation of their treatment plans. Although nonpharmacologic interventions are important components of a comprehensive chronic pain treatment plan, pharmacologic interventions invariably become central to the management of chronic pain in most patients. Thus, a thorough understanding of the pharmacology of analgesic drugs, particularly the pharmacology of opioids, is essential for optimal chronic pain management. For the reader's convenience, Box 5 lists websites that were reviewed by the authors and contain useful information on pain management. Thorough documentation of all patient encounters and all controlled substance prescriptions that are written is important. The use of pain consultants in the management of difficult cases is encouraged. Mental health consultants also should be

Box 5. Internet pain resources

If one enters "pain" in an internet search engine, such as Google, 19,000,000 webpages are listed. The following are among the most useful.

- American Pain Society (www.ampainsoc.org)
  The American Pain Society promotes education and research in pain management. It is one of the United States' leading resources for information on pain, such as pain management practice guidelines and policy statements regarding pain management issues. It is a leading resource for education on pain through its conferences and its monographs and books, which are available from this website.
- International Association for the Study of Pain (www.iasp-pain.org)
  The International Association for the Study of Pain is a multi-disciplinary international association that is dedicated to research and patient care on pain issues. It produces numerous publications on pain; all are available from this website.
- The Oxford Pain Internet Site (www.jr2.ox.ac.uk/bandolier/booth/painpag/)
  This website from Oxford University Press has a helpful "Clinical Bottom Line" site that covers a variety of pain issues.
- Canadian Pain Society (www.canadianpainsociety.ca)
  This website provides the recent Canadian Consortium on Pain Mechanisms, Diagnosis and Management's final report. Their goal is to improve the care of Canadians who are in pain through research and education.
- Medical College of Wisconsin (www.eperc.mcw.edu)
  This is a comprehensive website from the Medical College of Wisconsin with educational resources on pain and other end-of-life issues plus links to many other resources on pain management.
- The Dannemiller Memorial Educational Foundation (www.pain.com)
  This pharmaceutical industry–supported website is subtitled "a world of information on pain" and it delivers on its claim. There is not a more comprehensive site for current issues on pain management for providers and consumers.
- The National Institutes of Health Pain Consortium (painconsortium.nih.gov)
  This website from the national Institutes of Health lists ongoing clinical trials and research opportunities in pain. It also features links to recent publications in the area of pain research, as well as current news on pain issues.

considered in patients whose pain proves difficult to control because of the increased risk of psychologic morbidity in these patients.

Patients who are placed on chronic opioid therapy need to be counseled regarding issues of drug dependence and addiction at the initiation of opioid therapy. The prevalence of drug addictive behaviors in those without a previous substance abuse history is believed to be small; however, the occasional patient who demonstrates substance abuse behavior or non-compliance with the drug regimen must be confronted and the therapy discontinued. It is fundamental that a patient who receives long-term opioid treatment have all prescriptions filled at a single pharmacy, and that sufficient information about the treatment plan be shared with the pharmacist. This proactive step minimizes barriers that are related to the legal and regulatory oversight of opioid dispensing. It also ensures that the patient's entire drug regimen receives regular independent review for potential adverse effects and drug-drug interactions.

Summary

Managing surgical patients who have chronic pain that results from their surgical disease and its treatment can bring a new and rewarding dimension to surgical practice. Patients appreciate their surgeon's continued interest and involvement with them, and the surgeon can overcome a sense of abandonment that may accompany the discharge of a patient who is not healed fully. Patients who have chronic pain often understand that their pain will not disappear. That their surgeon will not disappear can help them to accept and live with their pain.

References

[1] Lee KF, Ray JB, Dunn GP. Chronic pain management and the surgical patient: barriers and opportunities. J Am Coll Surg 2001;193(6):689–701.
[2] Evans RM, Fine PG, Portenoy RK, editors. Pain management: management of persistent nonmalignant pain. Chicago (IL): American Medical Association; 2003.
[3] Daut RL, Cleeland CS, Flanery RC. Development of the Wisconsin Brief Pain Questionnaire to assess pain in cancer and other diseases. Pain 1983;17:197–210.
[4] Ferrell B, for the American Geriatrics Society's Panel on Pain. Management of persistent pain in older persons. J Am Geriatr Soc 2002;50:S205–24.
[5] Lawhorne L, Passerini J, Cranmer K, et al. Chronic pain management in the long-term care setting. Baltimore (MD): American Medical Directors Association; 1999.
[6] McIntosh H. Regulatory barriers take some blame for pain under treatment. J Natl Cancer Inst 1991;83:1202–4.
[7] Evans RM, Fine PG, Portenoy RK, editors. Pain management: overview of physiology, assessment and treatment. Chicago (IL): American Medical Association; 2003.
[8] Portenoy RK, Kanner RM, editors. Pain management: theory and practice. Philadelphia: FA Davis; 1996.
[9] Gamsa A. The role of psychological factors in chronic pain: a half century of study. Pain 1994;57:5–15.

[10] Jenson MP, McFarland CA. Increasing the reliability and validity of pain intensity measurement in chronic pain patients. Pain 1993;55:195–203.

[11] Banos JE, Bosch F, Canellas M, et al. Acceptability of visual analogue scales in the clinical setting: a comparison with verbal rating scales in postoperative pain. Methods Find Exp Clin Pharmacol 1989;11:123–7.

[12] Hirano PC, Laurent DD, Long K. Arthritis patient education studies, 1987–1991: a review of the literature. Patient Educ Couns 1994;24:9–54.

[13] NIH Technology Assessment Panel on Integration of Behavioral and Relaxation Approaches into the Treatment of Chronic Pain and Insomnia. Integration of behavioral and relaxation approaches into the treatment of chronic pain and insomnia. JAMA 1996; 276:313–8.

[14] Manchikanti L, Singh V, Kloth D, et al. Interventional techniques in the management of chronic pain part 2. Pain Physician 2001;4:24–96.

[15] Loitman JE. Pain management: beyond pharmacy to acupuncture and hypnosis. JAMA 2000;283:118–9.

[16] Cherkin DC, Sherman KJ, Deyo RA, et al. A review of the evidence for the effectiveness, safety, and cost of acupuncture, massage therapy, and spinal manipulation for back pain. Ann Int Med 2003;138:898–906.

[17] Chan F, Hung L, Suen B, et al. Celecoxib versus diclofenac and omeperazole in reducing the risk of recurrent ulcer bleeding in patients with arthritis. New Engl J Med 2002;347:2104–10.

[18] Ashburn MA, Lipman AG, Carr D, et al for the American Pain Society. Principles of analgesic use in the treatment of acute pain and cancer pain. 5th edition. Glenview (IL): American Pain Society; 2003.

[19] Hylek EM, Heiman H, Skates SJ, et al. Acetaminophen and other risk factors for excessive warfarin anticoagulation. JAMA 1998;279:657–62.

[20] Sindrup SH, Jensen TS. Efficacy of pharmacological treatments of neuropathic pain: an update and effect related to mechanism of drug action. Pain 1999;83:389–400.

[21] Thompson AR, Ray JB. The importance of opioid tolerance: a therapeutic paradox. J Am Coll Surg 2003;196(2):321–4.

[22] Ballantyne JC, Mao J. Opioid therapy for chronic pain. New Engl J Med 2003;349(20): 1943–51.

ELSEVIER
SAUNDERS

SURGICAL
CLINICS OF
NORTH AMERICA

Surg Clin N Am 85 (2005) 225–236

Neuropathic Pain: Implications for the Surgeon

Robert A. Milch, MD, FACS[a,b,*]

[a]State University of Buffalo, Buffalo, NY, USA
[b]The Center for Hospice and Palliative Care, 225 Como Park Boulevard,
Buffalo, NY 14227, USA

Pain management is the surgeon's stock-in-trade, whether accomplished by operative intervention or pharmacologic management. Although more commonly confronted with problems that are related to somatic or visceral nociceptive pain (ie, pain that is generated by tissue injury and resultant activation of nociceptive sensory axons), surgeons frequently encounter situations in which neuropathic pain symptoms predominate.

Although nociceptive pain typically is localized and diminishes with healing or elimination of the noxious stimulus, neuropathic pain may: (1) become chronic, even in the absence of a continuing stimulus; (2) serve no protective purpose in its chronicity; and (3) exact a significant toll on the patient's quality of life. Unrelieved, maladaptive symptoms (eg, anxiety, depression, insomnia) may ensue or sociopathic behaviors (eg, substance abuse) may follow. Although complex case management dealing with these psychosocial issues is afforded the best opportunity for success when overseen by specialists in comprehensive pain management centers [1,2], many straightforward and postoperative neuropathic pain syndromes are seen by surgeons. Thus, it behooves every practitioner to be familiar with the tools used and the underlying principles of their use. This article provides a brief overview of neuropathic pain—its mechanisms and situations a surgeon might encounter—and presents principles and recommendations for its primary pharmacologic management.

Understanding of neuropathic pain mechanisms led to the broad definition of it in 1994 by the International Association for the Study of Pain (IASP) as "pain initiated or caused by a primary lesion or dysfunction

* The Center for Hospice and Palliative Care, 225 Como Park Boulevard, Buffalo, NY 14227.
  E-mail address: rmilch@palliativecare.org

0039-6109/05/$ - see front matter © 2005 Elsevier Inc. All rights reserved.
doi:10.1016/j.suc.2004.12.001
surgical.theclinics.com

in the nervous system" [3]. De facto recognition of some of the unique aspects of neuropathic pain were reported first by a surgeon, Dr. Weir Mitchell, in his 1872 treatise, *Injuries of the Nerves and Their Consequences*, which described causalgia following Civil War wounds. Subsequent experience and studies led to a better understanding of the heterogeneous nature of the development and categorization of neuropathic pain types and syndromes which extend beyond the merely taxonomic and recognizes their clinical features and their mechanisms of generation [4,5].

Whatever the etiology, neuropathic pain is typified by three symptomatic features; each is present, to a greater or lesser degree, in most cases and is elucidated by careful history-taking and by eliciting verbal descriptors of the pain from the patient. First is dysesthesia, often described in terms of aching, cramping, or pressure, and, at times, as heat or "a hot poker" in the affected region. The second is intermittent, paroxysmal pain, which some-times is described as "electric shock" or lancinating; its appearance can be unprompted or brought on by tactile stimulation or movement. The last is allodynia, or an exaggerated perception of pain following a normally innocuous stimulus, or the experience of a cold stimulus as heat [6].

Several other symptoms are characteristic of neuropathic pain (Box 1). Hyperalgesia is an extremely painful response to an ordinarily mildly painful stimulus. In addition, there may be a summation phenomenon, wherein a single, bland mechanical stimulus does not induce pain, but continued or repeated stimulation evokes severe pain which often extends beyond the distribution of the injured nerve.

Finally, autonomic dysregulation may occur as a result of soft tissue trauma (reflex sympathetic dystrophy [RSD] or complex regional pain syndrome, type 1) or nerve injury (causalgia, or complex regional pain syndrome, type 2). The two syndromes are referred to as "sympathetically maintained pain"; the affected area or extremity shows sweating abnor-malities and vasomotor instability (eg, flushing, pallor). Over time, a limb may become edematous, the skin thin with loss of hair, and bones osteoporotic [7,8].

Neuropathic pain may be generated by peripheral or central mechanisms. Peripherally, compression or distortion of nervi nervora afferents in the connective tissue covering may produce nerve sheath pain. Axonal injury can stimulate nerve "sprouts" which may become generators of ectopic signals, particularly if they are trapped in scar tissue (neuromas) or if demyelination of the axon occurs (eg, Tinel's sign). Moreover, injured nerves may exhibit ephaptic transmission or cross-excitation of adjacent nerves that are responsible for perception of pain in near-by distributions, this often is referred to as "recruitment" [9].

Central generators of pain, so-called "deafferentation pain," may be caused by lesions in the central nervous system (eg, thalamic injury) or peripheral nervous system; the latter has changes that are induced first in dorsal horn nuclei thresholds of excitability. This phenomenon is

---

Box 1. Pain terms and definitions

Pain: An unpleasant sensory and emotional experience associated with actual or potential tissue damage, or described in terms of such

Neuropathic pain: Pain initiated or caused by a primary lesion or dysfunction in the nervous system

Central pain: Pain initiated or caused by a primary lesion or dysfunction in the central nervous system

Allodynia: Pain due to a stimulus that normally does not provoke pain

Causalgia: A syndrome of sustained burning pain, allodynia, and hyperpathia after a traumatic nerve lesion, often combined with vasomotor and sudomotor dysfunction and later trophic changes

Dysesthesia: An unpleasant, abnormal sensation, whether spontaneous or evoked

Hyperalgesia: An increased response to a stimulus that normally is painful

Hyperpathia: A painful syndrome that is characterized by an abnormally painful reaction to a stimulus, especially a repetitive stimulus, as well as an increased threshold

Hypoesthesia: Diminished sensation or numbness

Neuralgia: Pain in the distribution of a nerve or nerves

Neuropathy: A disturbance or pathologic change in a nerve; in one nerve, mononeuropathy; in several nerves, mononeuropathy multiplex; if diffuse and bilateral, polyneuropathy

Nociceptor: A receptor preferentially sensitive to a noxious stimulus

Noxious stimulus: One that is damaging to normal tissues

Paresthesia: An abnormal sensation, whether spontaneous or evoked

---

Data from Merskey H, Bogduk N, editors. Classification of chronic pain. 2nd edition. Seattle (WA): IASP Press; 1994.

---

particularly common when ongoing afferent stimulation, as with tumor encroachment or ischemia, results in hyperexcitability in regions of the dorsal horn, thalamus, and cortex. This causes sustained spontaneous and evoked pain, and explains, in part, the phenomena of allodynia, hyperpathia, and phantom limb syndrome [10].

Postsurgical neuropathic pain syndromes

Several pain syndromes are encountered frequently by oncologic surgeons. These include conditions that are associated with direct tumor encroachment (eg, cord compression or brachial and lumbar plexopathies), postradiation, and postchemotherapy syndromes. In addition, there are five common postoperative pain syndromes with which every surgeon should be familiar.

Postmastectomy and postaxillary lymph node dissection pain is seen in up to 10% of patients. Caused by trauma to the intercostobrachial cutaneous nerve (T1/T2), it is characterized by burning pain in the axilla, inner aspect of the upper arm, and adjacent chest wall and hypoesthesia in the affected area. Typically, it occurs in the immediate postoperative period, although it can occur months later. A tender trigger point may be palpable. Untreated, pain may lead to a "frozen shoulder" and significant functional disability. Its unique characteristics of pain usually differentiate it from the discomfort of later axillary tumor recurrence, which has a predominately somatic nociceptive quality [11].

Postthoracotomy pain is dysesthesia along the distribution of the intercostal nerve subjacent to a thoracotomy incision. Occurring soon postoperatively, it is likely from operative trauma. A later appearance may be due to tumor recurrence or neuroma formation; the latter mechanism is responsible for neuropathic pain that can occur in any incised wound that is adjacent to larger nerves (eg, ilio-inguinal neuropathy following hernia repair) [12].

Phantom limb pain is encountered most frequently when there has been prolonged preamputation extremity pain, that likely is caused by secondarily-induced central nervous system changes. It often has a lancinating, burning characteristic that may diminish over time, or be described as a pressure sensation in a limb that still is perceived to be present. When amputation is performed for malignant disease, its late occurrence may presage recurrent disease. Management is challenging, and no single approach is uniformly successful [13].

Amputation stump pain usually is from neuroma formation. It is elicited by mechanical stimulation of the stump or scar, and Tinel's sign may be demonstrable as a trigger point. It should be distinguished from phantom limb pain, in which the amputated extremity if perceived to be present. Pharmacologic therapy usually is effective in managing the former, whereas other interventions (revision, prosthesis adjustment, steroid or Botulinum injection) usually are required for the latter [14].

Postradical neck dissection pain is caused by trauma to transverse cervical nerves or the cervical plexus that result in dysesthetic pain in the neck and upper shoulder. It usually is apparent in the immediate postoperative period, although its later appearance may indicate tumor recurrence.

Management

Beydoun [15] suggested a mechanistically-based algorithm for approaching neuropathic pain. Consideration of invasive modalities, such as nerve blocks or surgical intervention (decompression, neuroaugmentation or ablative procedures, excision of neuromas) aside, pharmacologic management is the mainstay of treatment. Beyond the opioids, the drugs that are involved can be divided into two broad categories: membrane-stabilizing agents (certain anticonvulsants, corticosteroids, antiarrhythmics) and drugs that enhance dorsal horn inhibition (antidepressants, certain anticonvulsants, and antispasmodics) (Table 1).

Opioids

Unlike somatic or visceral nociceptive pain, neuropathic pain is less responsive to opioid analgesics [15–17]; although they provide a base for

Table 1
Selected drugs for neuropathic pain

Class	Generic name
Opioid	Morphine
	Oxycodone
	Hydromorphone
	Hydrocodone
	Fentanyl
	Methadone
Antidepressant	Amitryptiline
	Nortryptiline
	Desipramine
	Paroxetine
Anticonvulsant	Gabapentin
	Carbamazepine
	Oxcarbazepine
	Phenytoin
	Clonazepam
Topical agents	Capsaicin
	Lidocaine gel
	EMLA cream
GABAβ agonists	Baclofen
Local anesthetics (antiarrhythmics)	Lidocaine
	Mexilitene
α-2 Adrenergic agonists	Clonidine
	Phenoxybenzamine
	Prazosin
NMDA antagonists	Ketamine
	Dextromethorphan
Corticosteroids	Dexamethasone
	Prednisone

Abbreviations: GABAβ, γ-aminobutyric acid β; NMDA, N-methyl-D-aspartate.

management, high dosages may produce side effects that significantly affect the quality of life. To that end, management of neuropathic pain often entails empiric trials of various opioids; no one type is necessarily more effective than another. Coanalgesic or adjuvant drugs usually are necessary to achieve an acceptable level of pain control [18].

The opioid may be an immediate release formulation—which has peak activity at 1 to 2 hours, 4-hour duration, and is dosed on a regular basis—or a sustained release formulation, which is dosed orally every 8 to 24 hours (depending on the formulation) or transdermally every 48 to 72 hours. When low-dose opioid/nonopioid combinations are used, care must be taken to avoid toxic levels of the "add-on" drug—typically acetaminophen, which should be kept at levels less than 4 g/d.

Of the opioids, no one is more efficacious than another because they can be dose adjusted for equianalgesic effect (Table 2), and the individual patient's tolerance largely is idiosyncratic. Because of its pharmaceutical versatility (ie, available in the largest number of forms), morphine is the frequent drug of choice after need exceeds the relief that is provided by the opioid combination products. Whichever opioid is chosen, the principles of management of chronic pain need to be observed: regular dosing at intervals that are commensurate with the duration of action of the preparation, and provision of "rescue" or "breakthrough" dosages of an immediate release preparation (preferably the same drug) in an amount that roughly is equal to 15% to 20% of the total daily dose and given at 2-hour intervals as needed.

For several reasons, methadone is finding increasing use in the management of chronic pain, particularly neuropathic pain. In addition to producing analgesia centrally, it is an N-methyl-D-aspartate (NMDA) receptor inhibitor in the dorsal horn, where its effect is to diminish sensitivity to excitatory neurotransmitters that are responsible for many of the secondary qualities of neuropathic pain. A sustained-release opioid, it is the only one that is available in liquid form; this is a boon for patients who have dysphagia or are dependent on tube feedings. In addition, it is inexpensive. Although its use should be considered for many instances of neuropathic pain, because of its unique pharmacokinetics and pharmacodynamics, it can pose a significant risk for sedation and respiratory

Table 2
Equianalgesic dosing of opioids

Drug	Oral (mg)	Parenteral (mg)
Morphine	30	10
Hydrocodone	30	Not available
Hydromorphone	7.5	1.5
Oxycodone	30	Not available
Methadone	3–10	1.5–5
Fentanyl (transdermal) 25 mcg	60–90[a]	Not applicable

[a] Every 24 hours.

depression, particularly during dose escalation or in combination with other sedating drugs. It should be prescribed only by those who have experience in pain management (eg, pain or palliative care specialist).

Antidepressants

The tricyclic antidepressants (TCAs) (eg, amitriptyline, nortriptyline, desipramine) provide analgesia in several neuropathic pain syndromes that are characterized by continuous dysesthesias or intermittent lancinating pain [19]. Typically, the effective dosage is less than the antidepressant dosage, with an onset of action that varies from days to weeks as the dose is titrated upward to effect or to the limitations of side effects. The hypothesized mechanism by which TCAs act is complex; they seem to be selective inhibitors of norepinephrine or serotonin reuptake, and thus, help to modulate descending inhibitory pathways [20].

Although there is interindividual variability in responsiveness to the TCAs, all exhibit some degree of anticholinergic activity which may produce blurred vision, dry mouth, urinary retention, or precipitation of acute glaucoma. Patients who have significant heart disease (eg, arrhythmias, conduction disorders) probably should take other compounds. Somnolence also is common; for this reason, therapy usually is begun with nighttime dosing. Amitriptyline is the most widely studied TCA; dosing is begun at 10 mg, and if tolerated, is dosed upward to effect at 2- or 3-day intervals. Nortriptyline and desipramine also are effective with less sedation and fewer side effects reported.

Selective serotonin reuptake inhibitors have been studied as therapy for neuropathic pain. Although they lack the sedating and anticholinergic properties of TCAs, they have yielded inconsistent results in improving the pain syndromes [21]. Their combination with TCAs may allow smaller dosages of each to be used, with a more tolerable side effect profile.

Anticonvulsants

The specific mechanisms by which the anticonvulsants produce analgesia are not completely clear, although it likely is in large part from their suppression of paroxysmal discharges and overall neuronal hyperexcitability [22]. In larger series, they were most effective when treating paroxysmal or lancinating pain, although "newer" drugs (eg, gabapentin) also seem to be efficacious for continuous dysesthetic pain [23].

As with TCAs, there is large interindividual variation in response to the anticonvulsants. Gabapentin often is the first anticonvulsant that is chosen because of its favorable side effect profile and broad spectrum of efficacy. It usually is begun at a divided dose of 300 mg/d; in the absence of common side effects (eg, somnolence, nausea) it is titrated upward in 300-mg increments at 3-day intervals to effect, often at levels in excess of 1800 mg/d.

It must be used with extreme caution in the face of renal insufficiency and tapered when being discontinued [24].

Carbamazepine is effective in neuropathic pain management, but has a higher incidence of side effects—some serious. As with gabapentin, the common ones (eg, somnolence, nausea, dizziness) can be minimized with "low and slow" dosage titration. Bone marrow suppression, that is manifested as leukopenia, thrombocytopenia, or red cell aplasia, occurs in up to 1% of patients; ongoing monitoring of these parameters, as well as hepatic and renal function, is required. Severe dermatologic reactions with epidermal necrolysis or Steven-Johnson syndrome have been reported. Combination with other therapies that may have similar side effects or affect its metabolism can make its use problematic. Levels of carbamazepine need to be monitored to minimize the chance of toxicity. Oxcarbazepine is an analog of carbamazepine that similarly inhibits paroxysmal neuronal discharges and the release of excitatory neurotransmitters; thus, it modulates central and peripheral sensitization. It has not been studied widely, but seems to have an improved safety and side effect profile.

Clonazepam is a benzodiazepine that suppresses spike and wave neuronal discharges. It is effective in lancinating pain syndromes, but can be sedating; it must be used with caution in the presence of pre-existing seizure disorders, and can produce ataxia. Like all benzodiazepines, it must be tapered in discontinuation.

γ-Aminobutyric acidβ agonists

Baclofen, used for management of spasticity, also is useful for the treatment of lancinating and paroxysmal pain; it inhibits synaptic reflexes at the dorsal horn and other sites. Usually begun at a dosage of 5 mg, three times a day, slow upward titration to effect or a maximum of 90 mg/d minimizes the occurrence of common side effects (eg, sedation, dizziness, nausea). It must be tapered when being discontinued [25].

Corticosteroids

The mechanism by which corticosteroids produce analgesia in neuropathic pain are complex. They probably include reduction of peri-tumoral edema with subsequent diminution of pressure on nerves; a reduction of inflammatory mediators that can act as nociceptive sensitizers; and in certain malignant conditions, a decrease in tumor size or infiltration. Although there are few data to support the use of one corticosteroid over another, dexamethasone usually is preferred because of its potency equivalency and its small mineralocorticoid effect. In urgent situations (eg, spinal cord compression), dosages that are as large as 100 mg/d for 2 weeks have provided relief [26], whereas lower dose regimens (eg, 8 mg, twice daily) are effective in other plexopathies, such as Pancoast syndrome [27].

Antiarrhythmics (local anesthetics)

These drugs may be used systemically as second-line agents after antidepressants and anticonvulsants, or locally for trigger point injections or locoregional blockade [28]. Effective for continuous dysesthesias and lancinating pain, when applied locally they work by blocking sodium channels that are intrinsic for nerve conduction which results in a non-depolarizing block of transmission. Given systemically, they suppress firing of dorsal horn neurons and dorsal root ganglion cells.

Typically, trials of lidocaine infusions are begun at 2 to 4 mg/kg/30 min; relief may be prompt in onset and long-lasting. Mexilitene is an orally-active local anesthetic that usually is begun at a dosage of 150 mg, twice a day, given with food, and slowly titrated to a maximum of 900 mg a day. Adverse reactions tend to be dosage related and range from dizziness, tremor, and paresthesias at smaller dosages to seizures or encephalopathy at greater serum levels. In addition, serious cardiac events can be triggered, from conduction disturbances to frank myocardial depression and failure. Hence, serum levels must be monitored throughout therapy and patients who have pre-existing rhythm disturbances or cardiomyopathy usually are excluded from use [29].

α-2 Adrenergic agonists

These drugs reduce nociceptive input to the central nervous system by activating α-2 receptors in the spinal cord and brainstem. They also reduce sympathetic tone, and therefore, are useful in managing reflex sympathetic dystrophy and causalgia (sympathetically maintained syndromes). Generally resorted to after antidepressants, anticonvulsants, or oral local anesthetics have been used, clonidine is the agent that has been studied most extensively. Available for oral or transdermal administration, dosing is begun at a low dose (eg, 0.1 mg/d) and is titrated upward slowly. Common and troublesome side effects include orthostatic hypotension, dry mouth, and somnolence.

N-methyl-D-aspartate receptor antagonists

It is now known that the amino acids, aspartate and glutamate, are released by afferent neurons following noxious stimulation. In turn, these bind to the NMDA receptors in the spinal cord and brain and are key in the sensitization processes that are responsible for, and characteristic of, neuropathic pain. Agents that bind these receptors—and thus, prevent their activation by those circulating neurotransmitters—were effective in treating otherwise refractory neuropathic pain.

Ketamine is a dissociative general anesthetic that is used at subanesthetic levels for pain management. It can be trialed as a brief infusion over 1 hour (0.1–1.5 mg/kg) or as a continuous infusion at the same dose that is administered either intravenously or subcutaneously [30]. Upward titration must be done slowly and under close observation by experienced staff because there is a significant incidence of delirium, dysphoria, and hallucinations; some investigators recommend simultaneous administration of a benzodiazepine to decrease the emergence of these side effects. The effective oral dose may be substantively less than the parenteral dose [25,31].

Dextromethorphan has been inconsistently successful in helping to manage neuropathic pain [32]; however, it has far fewer side effects than ketamine, particularly in the frail or medically ill. Beginning at dosages of 60 mg per day, it can be titrated upward to effect or a maximum recommended dose of 1 gm daily.

Topical agents

For patients who are intolerant of systemically administered drugs, or for those who have predominately peripheral inciters of pain (eg, neuromas, locally traumatized peripheral nerves), topical agents may be helpful.

Capsaicin depletes noxious peptides (eg, substance P) in peripheral afferent neurons, which, in turn, are believed to activate nociceptive ganglia in the dorsal horn. Topically applied, it can produce local burning which, although it dissipates with repeated use, can be uncomfortable and require an analgesic for toleration [33]. It has proven efficacy in postmastectomy and postthoracotomy syndromes.

A eutectic mixture of local anesthetics (EMLA) cream is a combination of lidocaine and prilocaine. Applied in a thick layer and kept under an impermeable dressing, it is transdermally absorbed over 30 minutes and produces a local area of dense hypoesthesia. Similar effect may be obtained from 5% lidocaine gel or transdermal patches [34].

A word should be said for transcutaneous electrical nerve stimulation, a noninvasive topical therapy that essentially has no adverse effects and is beneficial in neuropathic pain management, particularly in peripherally maintained pain syndromes. The technique apparently "reorganizes" the afferent signals from fibers that ascend to the dorsal horn and inhibits pain perception and central reorganization [35].

Summary

Pharmacologic therapy for neuropathic pain is based on an evolving understanding of its underlying mechanisms, and often requires a patient, methodical sequence of trials that include the "four As": analgesics, antidepressants, anticonvulsants, and antiarrhythmics. Critical for success is a willingness to stay engaged with the patient to evolve a mutually acceptable plan and goals of care with realistic outcomes that emphasize symptom control and maximization of function. Such management is within the capabilities of surgeons for most patients, whereas the use of consultation and interdisciplinary supportive interventions from comprehensive pain management centers, if available, is helpful in more difficult cases.

References

[1] Flor H, Fydrich T, Turk DC. Efficacy of multidisciplinary pain treatment centers: a meta-analytic review. Pain 1992;49:221–30.
[2] Davies HT, Crombie IK, Macrae WA. Why use a pain clinic. Management of neurogenic pain before or after referral. J R Soc Med 1994;87:382–5.
[3] International Association for the Study of Pain. IASP pain terminology. Available at: http://www.halcyon.com/iasp. Accessed October 15, 2004.
[4] Woolf CJ, Mannion RJ. Neuropathic pain: etiology, symptoms, mechanisms, and management. Lancet 1999;353:1959–64.
[5] Attal N. Chronic neuropathic pain: mechanisms and treatment. Clin J Pain 2000;16: S118–23.
[6] Moulin DE. Neuropathic cancer pain: syndromes and clinical controversies. In: Bruera E, Portenoy RK, editors. Topics in palliative care, vol. 2. New York: Oxford University Press; 1998. p. 7–29.
[7] Merskey H, Bogduk N, editors. Classification of chronic pain. 2nd edition. Seattle (WA): IASP Press; 1994.
[8] Blumberg H, Janig W. Clinical manifestations of reflex sympathetic dystrophy and sympathetically maintained pain. In: Wall PD, Melzack R, editors. Textbook of pain. 3rd edition. New York: Churchill Livingstone; 1994.
[9] Devor M. The pathophysiology of damaged peripheral nerves. In: Wall PD, Melzack R, editors. Textbook of pain. 3rd edition. New York: Churchill Livingstone; 1994.
[10] Wall PD. Neuropathic pain and injured nerve: central mechanisms. Br Med Bull 1991;47: 631–43.
[11] Vecht CJ. Arm pain in the patient with breast cancer. J Pain Sympt Manage 1990;5:109–17.
[12] Kanner R, Martini M, Foley KM. Nature and incidence of postthoracotomy pain. Proc Am Soc Clin Oncol 1982;1:152.
[13] Jensen TS, Rasmussen P. Phantom pain and other phenomena after amputation. In: Wall PD, Melzack R, editors. Textbook of pain. 3rd edition. New York: Churchill Livingstone; 1994.
[14] Kern U, Martin C, Muller H. Botulinum toxin type A influences stump pain after limb amputations. J Pain Symptom Manage 2003;26(6):1069–70.
[15] Beydoun A. Neuropathic pain: from mechanisms to treatment strategies. J Pain Symptom Manage 2003;25:5S.
[16] Portenoy RK, Forbes K, Lussier D, et al. Difficult pain problems: an integrated approach. In: Doyle D, Hanks G, Cherny N, et al, editors. Oxford textbook of palliative medicine. 3rd edition. Oxford (UK): Oxford University Press; 1998. p. 438–58.
[17] Jadad AR. Opioids in the treatment of neuropathic pain: a systematic review of controlled clinical trials. In: Bruera E, Portenoy RK, editors. Topics in palliative care, vol. 2. New York: Oxford University Press; 1998.
[18] Portenoy RK. Issues in the management of neuropathic pain. In: Basbaum A, Besson JM, editors. Towards a new pharmacotherapy of pain. New York: John Wiley and Sons; 1991.
[19] Onghena P, Van Houdenhove B. Antidepressant induced analgesia in chronic non-malignant pain: a meta-analysis of 39 placebo controlled studies. Pain 1992;49:205–19.
[20] Watson CP. The treatment of neuropathic pain: antidepressants and opioids. Clinic J Pain 2000;16(2 Suppl):49–55.
[21] Edwards JG, Anderson I. Systematic review and guide to selection of selective serotonin reuptake inhibitors. Drugs 1999;57:507–33.

[22] Tremont-Lukats IW, Megeff C, Backonja MM. Anticonvulsants for neuropathic pain syndromes: mechanisms of action and place in therapy. Drugs 2000;60:1029–52.

[23] McQuay HJ, Carroll D, Jadad AR. Anticonvulsant drugs for the management of pain: a systematic review. BMJ 1995;311:1047–52.

[24] Mosby's Drug Consult. 15th edition. St. Louis (MO): Mosby Inc; 2005. Available at: http://online.statref.com. Accessed on January 15, 2005.

[25] Hewitt DJ, Portenoy RK. Adjuvant drugs for neuropathic cancer pain. In: Bruera E, Portenoy RK, editors. Topics in palliative care, vol. 2. New York: Oxford University Press; 1998.

[26] Vecht J, Haaxma-Reiche H, van Putten W, et al. Initial bolus of conventional versus high-dose dexamethasone in metastatic spinal cord compression. Neurology 1989;39:1255–7.

[27] Ettinger AB, Portenoy RK. The use of corticosteroids in the treatment of symptoms associated with cancer. J Pain Symptom Manage 1988;3:99–103.

[28] Covino BG. Local anesthetics. In: Ferrante FM, VadeBoncouer TR, editors. Postoperative pain management. New York: Churchill Livingstone; 1993. p. 211–53.

[29] Campbell RWF. Mexilitene. N Engl J Med 1987;3116:29–34.

[30] Backonja M, Arndt G, Gombar KA, et al. Response of chronic neuropathic pain syndromes to ketamine: a preliminary study. Pain 1994;56:51–7.

[31] Fisher K, Hagen NA. Analgesic effect of oral ketamine in chronic neuropathic pain of spinal origin: a case report. J Pain Symptom Manage 1999;18(1):61–6.

[32] McQuay HJ, Carroll D, Jadad AR, et al. Dextromethorphan for the treatment of neuropathic pain: a double blind randomized controlled crossover trial. Pain 1994;59:127–33.

[33] Dubner R. Topical capsaicin therapy for neuropathic pain. Pain 1991;47:247–8.

[34] Rowbotham MC, Davies PS, Fields HL. Topical lidocaine gel relieves postherpetic neuralgia. Ann Neurol 1995;37:246–53.

[35] Walsh DM. TENS physiological principles and stimulation parameters: the clinical application of TENS and related theory. Edinburgh (Scotland): Churchill Livingstone; 1997.

SURGICAL
CLINICS OF
NORTH AMERICA

Surg Clin N Am 85 (2005) 237–255

Common Symptoms in Advanced Cancer

Ruth L. Lagman, MD, MPH*,
Mellar P. Davis, MD, FCCP,
Susan B. LeGrand, MD, FACP,
Declan Walsh, MSc, FACP, FRCP (Edin)

*The Harry R. Horvitz Center for Palliative Medicine,
Cleveland Clinic Taussig Cancer Center, The Cleveland Clinic Foundation,
9500 Euclid Avenue, M76 Cleveland, OH 44195, USA*

Anorexia and cachexia

Introduction

Anorexia and cachexia are a major cause of morbidity and mortality in advanced cancer. Involuntarily weight loss is characteristic of solid tumors, particularly those that are derived from foregut organs. Eighty percent of patients who have upper gastrointestinal cancers and 60% of patients who have lung cancer have lost a substantial amount of weight at diagnosis [1,2]. In contrast, hematologic malignancies, breast cancer, and hindgut malignancies are not associated with anorexia and cachexia or develop symptoms and signs late in the course of illness [3]. Cachexia is more common in children and the elderly and becomes more evident with advanced stages; cachexia is present in 50% of patients who have active cancer and 80% of patients at the time of death [1]. Patients who have cancer who experience 5% or more weight loss have a significantly shorter survival than those who do not have weight loss [1]. Weight loss decreases the tolerance to radiation, chemotherapy and surgery. Cachexia reduces performance status and determines quality of life to a greater extent than pain in advanced cancer [4]. The detrimental effects of catabolism that are associated with cachexia are responsible for 20% of cancer deaths [1,2].

Anorexia occurs in advanced cancer, despite an increased need for calories. Cancer disengages the normal balance between appetite signals and

The Harry R. Horvitz Center for Palliative Medicine is a World Health Organization Demonstration Project. Available at: http://www.clevelandclinic.org/palliative.

* Corresponding author.
E-mail address: lagmanr@ccf.org (R.L. Lagman).

energy expenditures [5]. Anorexia, as measured by dietary intake, does not correlate well with the degree of weight loss. Weight loss can be precipitous, despite a normal appetite [5–8]. Anorexia in cancer may be a general loss of appetite, early satiety, altered food preferences, or a combination of these. There is a distinct difference in the proposed pathophysiology between cancer and anorexia such that anorexia and cachexia should not be considered synonymous although they overlap in frequency.

Pathophysiology of cachexia and anorexia

Cachexia

Cachexia is a systemic inflammatory response that is caused by host-generated cytokines; tumor-derived cytokines; or specific (unique) cachexins that detrimentally alter carbohydrate, lipid, and protein metabolism. Cachexia differs from starvation. Clinically, cachexia must be differentiated from secondary caloric deprivation that is caused by mechanical interference of food absorption (eg, bowel obstruction, dysphagia, malabsorption, nausea, vomiting). Caloric deprivation will respond to aggressive nutritional support in the form of parenteral nutrition, whereas cachexia will not [6].

Glucose used by tumors is inefficient because most cancers are hypoxic and are unable to metabolize glucose fully to CO_2. Tumors use glucose as a primary source of energy and generate a large amount of lactate which is converted to glucose in the liver by way of the Cori cycle [9–11]. Fifty percent of glucose turnover in advanced cancer is through the Cori cycle; this is 20% in normal individuals. In addition, alanine from proteolysis and glycerol from lipolysis are diverted to glucose by the liver [9,11,12]. The generation of glucose from lactate in the process of gluconeogenesis requires six ATP molecules which is energy inefficient; this accounts for some of the high resting energy expenditures in cancer [9].

Resting energy expenditures are increased in cancer, particularly when energy expenditures are corrected for lean body mass rather than body mass index. Men have higher resting energy expenditures than women. Although resting energy expenditures are increased, total energy expenditures can be unchanged as a result of a patient-adapted sedentary existence [13–15]. Increased sympathetic activity in cancer causes increased resting energy expenditures [16]. Recently discovered uncoupling proteins ($UCP_{1,2,3,4}$) were found to increase brown adipose tissue, liver, and skeletal muscle heat generation at the cost of stored energy in the form of ATP [17]. Uncoupling proteins divert electrons from ATP production in the mitochondrion in favor of thermogenesis and increased resting energy expenditures [18]. A tumor-specific cachexin, now known as a zinc-α2-glycoprotein, identical to the lipid mobilizing factor (LMF), increases uncoupling proteins in adipose tissue and skeletal muscle [19]. Several other mediators are responsible for increased resting energy expenditures in advanced cancer, including increased neurohumoral agonists, cytokines, and tumor-specific cachexins.

Patients who have cancer have increased insulin resistance that leads to increased lipolysis and hyperlipidemia that is unresponsive to glucose infusions [12,20–23]. Glycerol clearance also is reduced [24]. Several factors seem to be responsible for increased lipolysis and reduced lipid anabolism that are associated with cancer. Increased sympathetic activity is responsible, in part, for lipolysis [25,26]. The cytokines, leukemia inhibitory factor and tumor necrosis factor (TNF), decrease lipoprotein lipase activity; this reduces triglyceride clearance from the blood and blocks lipid storage in adipocytes [27]. A second tumor-specific cachexin, anemia-inducing substance, increased lipolysis in patients who had ovarian cancer [28,29]. Interferons also increase in advanced cancer and decrease lipoprotein lipase activity and triglyceride clearance [30]. Finally, LMF also induces lipolysis through β-adrenoreceptors on adipocytes [31,32]. As with altered carbohydrate metabolism, multiple factors are responsible for altered lipid metabolism.

Skeletal muscle wasting occurs as a result of the up-regulation of the ubiquitin–proteasome-dependent pathway [33]. Actin and myosin are targeted for catabolism by proteasomes. Other factors that lead to proteolysis include certain carrier proteins, transcription factors, and nuclear factor kappaB (NF-κB) that up-regulate proteasomes and reduced protein synthesis [34]. Hormone mediators of muscle catabolism include corticosteroids, which increase the components of proteasomes. TNF prevents production of new muscle through up-regulation of the transcription factor, NFκB. Tumor-specific proteolysis is induced by proteolysis-inducing factor, which induces proteasome production through the prostaglandin, hydroeicosatetraenoic acid (15-HETE) [35].

Appetite signals are blunted in cancer. The normal hunger signal that is derived from neuropeptide Y within the hypothalamus is qualitatively and quantitatively diminished in cancer, whereas the satiety signals that are generated by melacortins are amplified. Central mediators of anorexia are interleukin-1, serotonin, and TNF [5].

Assessment

Assessment of nutritional status requires a dietary history, review of systems (focused particularly on gastrointestinal symptoms), physical examination, biochemistry (albumin, pre-albumin, C-reactive protein), anthropometric measurements, and bioelectric impedance [36].

At least three quality-of-life instruments are validated in the assessment of anorexia and cachexia. They are: (1) Functional Assessment of Anorexia/ Cachexia Therapy, (2) Subjective Global Assessment, and (3) Bristol-Myers Anorexia/Cachexia Recovery Instrument [37–39]. Bioelectric impedance measures tissue electronic resistance (nonlean body mass) and capacitance (lean body mass) and accurately measures cachexia (and sarcopenia) better than body mass index and anthropometric measurements [36,40–42]. Overall nutritional assessment should be multi-dimensional if it is to reflect clinical reality. Treatment outcomes that use only one or two dimensions of assessment (body mass index, appetite, or anthropometric measurements) inaccurately gauge for clinical benefit and interventions.

Management

Management of anorexia and cachexia requires initial treatment of reversible causes for weight loss, such as bowel obstruction, dysphagia, and mucositis. Appetite stimulants, anticytokines, and antitumor cachexins may be important in relieving anorexia and forestalling or reversing weight loss, particularly if used in combination. The provision of calories is a necessity when secondary causes for weight loss are evident. Nutritional support, in the form of enteral or parenteral nutrition, has limited benefit in cachexia. Nutritional support does not reverse the catabolic metabolism of cachexia in advanced cancer [43,44]. Appetite stimulants, including include progesterones and corticosteroids, have some symptom benefit by evidence-based studies [45–48]. Corticosteroids accelerate muscle wasting and progesterones increase body fat, rather than lean body mass [49]. Neither one significantly influences quality of life.

Agents that reverse the inflammatory response that is caused by the host or tumor-specific cachexin have some potential for improving appetite and reversing catabolism [50]. Anticachexins include eicosapentaenoic acid, melatonin, thalidomide, nonsteroidal anti-inflammatory drugs, anabolic steroids, and 5 deoxy-5-fluorouridine [1,45,51]. In particular, eicosapentaenoic acid has promise as demonstrated in phase II studies. A dose-finding phase I study has been performed [52–54]; however, a recently completed, randomized clinical trial of low-dose eicosapentaenoic acid in a nutritional supplement found no clinical benefit. Further trials that use higher doses, based on phase I studies, will be needed to appreciate fully the benefits of eicosapentaenoic acid or confirm the lack of benefit. Other anticytokines that should be studied are soluble interleukin-6 receptor; soluble TNF receptor; and interleukin-4, -10, -12, and -15.

Dyspnea

Dyspnea, a subjective sense of difficulty breathing, remains a troubling symptom in advanced cancer. In a multi-national study that evaluated the practice of terminal sedation, 25% to 53% of those who required sedation did so for reasons of dyspnea [55]. Treatment of the underlying cause is the mainstay of therapy; however, as disease progression occurs, usual interventions become too burdensome or a different strategy may be needed.

Pathophysiology

Dyspnea is subjective and has a multi-dimensional physical, emotional, and social component. There are no tests (eg, oximetry, pulmonary function test, chest radiograph, arterial blood gas) that correlate with the presence or severity. It is whatever the patient says it is. A patient who has a normal respiratory rate, normal blood gas, and a normal chest radiograph may be dyspneic. Studies of the correlates of dyspnea found that weakness of the respiratory muscles plays a significant role [56–58]. Nevertheless, abnormalities often are identified that can be addressed specifically. In the setting of malignancy, these can be divided into complications of the disease, complications of therapy, and comorbid conditions. One also can consider pathology by organ system, such as: (1) pulmonary compromise that are due to pneumonia, primary or metastatic malignancy, pleural effusions, embolus and restrictive defects that are due to chest wall or intercostal and diaphragm muscle dysfunction; (2) cardiac abnormalities (eg, congestive heart failure, myocardial infarction, tamponade, arrhythmia); and (3) other factors (eg, anemia, cachexia).

Assessment

The goals of care should guide the evaluation. The first step is a careful history that identifies the time course (sudden versus progressive), exacerbating or relieving factors (eg, positional change, medications), associated symptoms (cough, fever, pain), and intensity. Although multidimensional scales exist, visual analog scales and numeric rating scales have been validated [59]. A 5-point verbal rating scale also has been validated using the terms none, mild, moderate, severe, and horrible [60]. The most readily treated causes that are identified in advanced disease are hypoxemia, anemia, and bronchospasm [57]. In most circumstances, oximetry and complete blood count or hematocrit should be done. In the in-patient setting, a chest radiograph also is indicated in all but the actively dying.

Management

Management of the underlying cause is beyond the scope of this article; therefore, we only will address the symptomatic approaches. As with all other symptoms, treatment of the sensation should be initiated even when detailed evaluation and aggressive interventions are planned. There is no need to wait for results to begin the therapies that are outlined below. Nonpharmacologic interventions, such as fans and positioning, also should be considered.

Opioids

The primary symptomatic therapy for dyspnea is morphine or an alternative opioid. A Cochrane review found evidence to support their use in the setting of advanced cancer [61]. In the naïve, starting doses should be 5 mg orally or 1 mg parentally (intravenous or subcutaneous routes). A continuous infusion that starts at 0.5 mg/hr is reasonable for rest dyspnea rather than episodic symptoms. If "as needed" dosing is begun, then a continuous infusion or oral sustained-release medications should be used if frequent dosing is required. Morphine is then titrated to relief and at the same time, monitoring toxicity. Respiratory depression generally is not seen with careful titration. Medications to treat side effects of opioids, particularly constipation, should be started simultaneously. Nebulized morphine has been controversial and controlled trials have not confirmed benefit [8]; however, a recently published abstract found comparable efficacy with less toxicity when compared with the subcutaneous route [62].

Corticosteroids

There are no controlled trials on the role of corticosteroids in the management of dyspnea in advanced disease. They are used particularly in the setting of lymphangitic spread, superior vena cava syndrome, or pulmonary toxicity from chemotherapy or radiation. Dosing is not standard but we typically use 4 mg to 8 mg by mouth at 8 AM and noon and continue if beneficial.

Bronchodilators

Unsuspected bronchospasm is identified commonly with pulmonary function testing in patients who have advanced disease [57,63]. Because this testing may be difficult for these individuals, a therapeutic trial of bronchodilators is reasonable. They should be discontinued if there is no symptomatic benefit.

Anxiolytics

The relationship of anxiety and dyspnea is difficult to clarify. There is a definite correlation, but cause and effect are less clear [56,64]. Therefore, the role of benzodiazepines is poorly defined. A recent trial of oral midazolam and oral morphine found equal efficacy but more side effects in the group that was given morphine [65]. Chlorpromazine has synergistic effects with morphine and also can be used for palliative sedation as a single agent, if indicated [66].

Oxygen

The role of oxygen is controversial. It is considered to be a benign intervention yet it limits mobility and may be irritating, cause nasal bleeding, and interfere with eating and conversation if delivered by ventimask. There was no symptomatic benefit in a controlled, blinded trial that involved nonhypoxic patients [67]. Because dyspnea does not correlate with oxygen levels, routine use in nonhypoxic patients is not justified. The placebo effect of oxygen may be beneficial in nonhypoxic patients, although other measures should be used before oxygen in the hypoxic patient (O_2 saturation less than 89%) to prevent cardiopulmonary decompensation by minimizing pulmonary hypertension.

Delirium

Overview

Delirium is a common and complex problem in palliative medicine. In a prospective study, 42% of patients were delirious on admission, 45% developed it during the admission, and 88% were delirious at death [68]. Frequently, it is unrecognized and undertreated yet it creates significant distress for patients who may remember the event, particularly if the delirium is mild or moderate [69]. Distress is even greater for families and nurses who provide bedside care.

Diagnosis

Delirium presents in three forms: (1) hyperactive—the easily recognized agitated, potentially aggressive patient; (2) hypoactive—that may be mistaken for depression and, therefore, often missed; or (3) mixed. The diagnosis is made using the *Diagnostic and Statistical Manual of Mental Disorders, Fourth Edition* criteria that has four key elements:

Disturbance in consciousness
    Reduced clarity of environmental awareness
    Impaired ability to focus
    Impaired ability to shift attention
Change in cognition not better explained by pre-existing, established, evolving dementia
    Memory impairment
    Disorientation
    Language disturbance
    Perceptual disturbance
Evolves over a short period of time
    Hours to days
    Fluctuates during the course of the day
    Evidence that the disturbance is caused by physiologic consequences of a general medical condition

There are multiple, validated tools that can be used for screening, such as the Delirium Rating Scale, The Confusion Assessment Method, or the Mini-Mental Status Examination. Whichever method is chosen, testing should be done on admission and then assessed periodically, particularly after medication changes [70].

Pathophysiology

Research suggests that disturbances of various neurotransmitters, particularly acetylcholine, but also dopamine and serotonin, may underlie delirium. The symptoms may reflect a final common pathway of multiple factors

[71]. Patient factors may predispose to the development of delirium, such as advanced age, pre-existing cognitive dysfunction, hearing or visual dysfunction, metabolic or nutritional deficits, and unfamiliar surroundings. Causative factors include medications, infections, surgery, metabolic abnormalities, hypoxemia, pain, withdrawal from medications/alcohol, physical restraints, and others [72]. In the palliative medicine population, the most common causes that were identified were medications, infection, and central nervous system malignancy [68]. Most, if not all medications that are prescribed frequently for symptom management have delirium as a potential toxicity.

If delirium is recognized in a patient, physicians need to evaluate the ability of patients to make decisions. This is one of the more difficult decisions that faces a palliative medicine specialist. Terminal delirium by definition is irreversible, and unfortunately, has no unique identifying features that separate it from reversible delirium. Only in hindsight will one know if delirium was reversible. The goals of treatment, therefore, need to be determined by the attending physician and family. Is it control of the agitation that may require sedation, or an aggressive evaluation that looks for reversible causes and specific treatment of the underlying cause for delirium? The goals of managing delirium should be based upon pre-event performance status, quality of life, and life expectancy. Would the person tolerate treatment of brain metastases if identified? Would treatment of an infection, if present, be indicated in light of the projected survival and preinfection quality of life?

The first step in evaluation of delirium is a careful history. The onset of delirium with a new event, such as a new medication or fever, may be helpful. Identifying the time course can identify any medication adjustments that may have led to the cognitive changes. If appropriate, laboratory testing should include complete blood count and chemistries; renal and hepatic function should be done. Oximetry is reasonable because the addition of oxygen is a simple intervention. CT scans or MRI of brain should be considered, depending on the goals of care and prognosis. If infection is suspected, empiric antibiotics are reasonable. Some investigators recommend a time-limited trial of fluid resuscitation. although the benefits are mixed [73]. Regardless of what type of evaluation is planned, treatment of agitation and hallucinations should begin immediately.

Treatment

The treatment of delirium involves treatment of the underlying cause, if appropriate, and management of the symptom with neuroleptic agents, such as haloperidol [70]. Olanzapine, respiridone, and quetiapine also have been used; however, they do not have parenteral forms in the United States [74–76]. These medications have proven efficacy in hyper- and hypoactive delirium. Although benzodiazepines are the medication of choice in the setting of withdrawal from substances, they rarely should be used in most patients who have delirium, yet they are commonly prescribed. In a small, randomized, controlled trial of haloperidol, chlorpromazine, and lorazepam in HIV-positive patients who had delirium, the lorazepam arm was closed secondary to lack of efficacy and worsening of symptoms in all six patients who were randomized to receive it [77]. For terminal sedation, medications, such as chlorpromazine, phenobarbital, and midazolam, have been used with success [78].

Nausea and vomiting

Nausea and vomiting occur commonly in patients who have advanced illness. Their prevalence varies widely; however, approximately 60% to 70% will experience nausea and 30% will experience vomiting in the last weeks of life [79–81]. Nausea is a subjective, unpleasant sensation of wanting to vomit. Vomiting is the forceful expulsion of gastric contents, whereas retching is an attempt to bring up something accompanied by contractions of the abdominal and intestinal muscles [82,83]. Most empiric research is focused on chemotherapy-induced nausea and vomiting. There is a scarcity of data on nausea and vomiting from other causes.

Pathophysiology

Afferent pathways in the central nervous system and gut connect to the vomiting center through neurotransmitters that are located in the nucleus of the tractus solitarius and reticular formation of the medulla. These afferent pathways include: (1) chemoreceptor trigger zone (CTZ) that is located in the fourth ventricle with dopamine (D_2), serotonin ($5HT_3$), acetylcholine (ACH), and neurokinin-1 (NK-1) receptors; (2) gastrointestinal tract with D_2, ACH, and $5HT_3$ receptors; (3) vestibulocochlear nerve (histamine and ACH) and; (4) cortex [83,84]. Understanding the underlying pathophysiology of nausea and vomiting, the knowledge of neural pathways, and drug pharmacology is paramount because these will lead to an appropriate choice of drugs and minimize side effects. A combination of these neural pathways may be responsible for nausea and vomiting.

Etiology

The common causes of nausea and vomiting in advanced illness include metabolic abnormalities (hepatic failure, hypercalcemia, hyponatremia, uremia); brain metastases, with increased intracranial pressure; bowel obstruction; chemotherapy; radiation therapy; constipation; and medications (antibiotics, nonsteroidal anti-inflammatory drugs, opioids, vitamin/mineral supplements). Emotional distress, such as anxiety, can cause nausea

[85,86]. A significant number of individuals who have advanced disease have pain and are treated with opioids. The CTZ and the vomiting center have opioid receptors that are emetogenic [83].

Assessment

A detailed history and physical examination are essential. Early morning headaches with nausea and vomiting are common with brain metastases, particularly those that are located in the cerebellum. Large volume emesis with colic and abdominal pain is associated with bowel obstruction. Nausea and vomiting with movement denotes vestibular dysfunction or mesenteric metastases. For individuals who are on several medications for multiple symptoms, an offending medication—commonly opioids and antibiotics—is a common cause. Laboratory tests, radiographic examinations, CT, and MRI help to confirm abnormalities that are suspected on history and physical examination.

Treatment

D_2 antagonists, including phenothiazines (chlorpromazine, prochorper-azine, promethazine) and butyrophenones (haloperidol), are the principal drug classes that are used to treat nausea. Phenothiazines are more sedating which often limits their use, whereas haloperidol is less sedating [83,84]. Olanzapine, a new atypical antipsychotic, is a dopamine and serotonin antagonist and is useful in refractory nausea and vomiting [87].

Metoclopramide, a substituted benzamide, is a dopamine antagonist and a serotonin antagonist at high dosages (ie, more than 120 mg/day). Akathisia and extrapyramidal symptoms may occur and may not be dose related [83]. Another prokinetic, domperidone, has antidopaminergic activity; it does not cause sedation and extrapyramidal symptoms because it does not cross the blood–brain barrier.

Antihistamines, like meclizine and cyclizine, are used to treat nausea and vomiting secondary to motion sickness, but also are ancillary drugs for bowel obstruction or nausea that are associated with brain metastases. The most common side effect is drowsiness. Dronabinol, a cannabinoid, acts on central cannabinoid receptors 1 and peripheral cannabinoid receptors 2, which reduces gastrointestinal motility and nausea. Its main side effect is mood changes, principally dysphoria, in the elderly [88].

$5HT_3$ receptor antagonists (granisetron, ondansetron, dolasetron) are effective in nausea and vomiting that are caused by chemotherapy and radiation [89]. The NK_1 receptor antagonist, aprepitant, when combined with ondansetron and dexamethasone is even more effective for the acute and delayed phases of chemotherapy [90]. Aprepitant relieves delayed nausea and vomiting due to chemotherapy to a greater extent than $5HT_3$ receptor antagonists.

Octreotide relieves nausea, vomiting, and cramping from malignant bowel obstruction. [83] It also decreases gastrointestinal secretions that are generated as a result of having a bowel obstruction.

Palliative venting procedures, such as gastrostomy, percutaneous endoscopic gastromy (PEG) [91], or percutaneous transesophageal gastrotubing (PTEG) [92], are surgical interventions that relieve symptoms from malignant bowel obstruction that are refractory to medications.

Fatigue

The subjective symptom of fatigue—often referred to by patients as feeling tired, weary, or having a lack of energy—is among the most common symptoms in advanced cancer. It is reported by 60% to 90% of patients [93]. The Fatigue Practice Guidelines Panel defines cancer-related fatigue "as an unusual, persistent, subjective sense of tiredness related to cancer or cancer treatment that interferes with usual functioning" [94].

Pathophysiology

The metabolic process that is responsible for causing fatigue is unknown. It is speculated that fatigue may be the end-result combination of different abnormal metabolic pathways [95]. Because cachexia and fatigue often occur together, the role of cytokines (TNF and interleukins) in the pathogenesis of fatigue has been proposed [96]; however, this remains to be proved.

Etiology

Fatigue in patients who have advanced cancer frequently is a result of multiple factors. These include cancer treatment modalities (chemotherapy/ radiation), paraneoplastic syndromes, comorbid illnesses (hypothyroidism, congestive heart failure), cachexia and severe muscle wasting, anemia, sleep disorders, psychologic factors (anxiety/depression), other symptoms of advanced cancer (pain, dyspnea, nausea), and medications (narcotic analgesics).

Assessment

Because fatigue is highly subjective, a thorough history of its temporal nature, exacerbating factors, and effect on overall quality of life need to be assessed. Patients do not often volunteer fatigue as a symptom, and therefore, physicians need to ask the patient if it is present.

Assessment instruments include unidimensional scales (eg, Fatigue Severity Scale [97], the Rhoten Fatigue Scale [98], and the Visual Analogue/ Numerical Rating Scale [99]). Examples of multi-dimensional scales include the Brief Fatigue Inventory [100], Piper Fatigue Self Report Scale [101], and the Cancer Fatigue Scale [102]. Performance status scales include the Edmonton Functional Assessment Test [103] and the Karnofsky Performance Status [104].

Treatment

Often, a treatable cause of fatigue is identified. Treatment of pain, depression, insomnia, and anemia (blood transfusion and erythropoietin) can reduce fatigue significantly. Metabolic and endocrine disorders can cause fatigue, and if treated, may improve performance status. Patient education improves the patient's ability to cope with their fatigue [99].

The best nonpharmacologic treatment to improve fatigue is moderate aerobic repetitive exercise [105,106]. The exercise regimen that is implemented has to be individualized and needs to be performed consistently to have optimal benefits [95]. Other alternative modes of treatment include relaxation, distraction, and guided imagery as well as restorative activities, such as gardening, meditation, or prayer.

The psychostimulant, methylphenidate, improves fatigue and depression [107]. Another psychostimulant, modafinil, improved fatigue in patients who had multiple sclerosis but has not been tested in patients who have cancer [108]. Other drugs diminish fatigue, including methylprednisolone [109] and megestrol acetate [110]. In time, however, corticosteroids will increase skeletal muscle proteolysis and lower extremity weakness. Megestrol acetate also can produce cushingoid-like side effects.

Constipation

The prevalence of constipation in patients who have advanced illness is approximately 40% [80]; the greatest prevalence occurs in the opioid-treated population [111]. A study of 498 terminally ill patients who had cancer showed that laxatives were administered to 87% of patients who were on strong opioids, 74% of patients who were on weak opioids, and 64% of patients who were not taking any narcotics [112]. Although opioid administration is used often for pain by patients who have advanced illness, other factors may play a role in the prevalence of constipation.

Pathophysiology

The general population in North America will describe "normal" bowel movements as anywhere from three times a day to three times a week. Because constipation is a symptom, the relative use of the term makes it harder to define. The Rome criteria was developed for a diagnosis of constipation. To meet the criteria, in the past 3 months, patients should have: (1) straining, (2) hard stools, (3) incomplete evacuation, (4) anorectal blockage, (5) needed disimpaction, and (6) less than three bowel movements in a week. In addition, loose stools should not be present and the criteria for irritable bowel syndrome is not met.

Normal bowel movement is mediated by the central and peripheral nervous system, hormones, and reflexes that are unique to the gastrointestinal system [113]. The peripheral nervous system, which is mediated by the sympathetic and parasympathetic nerves, controls colonic motility, retrocollic reflexes, and relaxation and contraction of the anal sphincter. The urge to defecate and the process of defecation itself is mediated partially by the central nervous system. Gastrointestinal hormone physiology is controlled by the endocrine, paracrine, and various neural pathways [114].

Etiology

The causes of constipation are varied and range from reversible, correctable etiologies to irreversible factors that include: (1) neurologic abnormalities (spinal cord lesions, autonomic neuropathy), (2) metabolic disorders (hypokalemia, hypercalcemia, uremia, diabetes mellitus), (3) structural abnormalities (fibrosis, obstruction), and (4) drugs (antihypertensives, opioids, antidepressants, diuretics, vitamin and mineral supplements).

Assessment

Although a decrease in the frequency of bowel movement often is reported by patients who have constipation, other clinical symptoms may include bloating, abdominal fullness, nausea, vomiting, diarrhea, and abdominal pain. The initial history taking should include a thorough review of bowel movement pattern, comorbid illnesses, and the patient's medications. Physical examination should focus on palpable abdominal masses and fecal impaction through a rectal examination. An abdominal radiograph and routine electrolytes should complete the initial diagnostic work-up. If necessary, further diagnostic work-up can be added as indicated.

Treatment

Nonpharmacologic maneuvers to prevent constipation include increased fluid intake, increased physical activity, and attempting to maintain regular bowel movements at the same time each day. Increasing dietary fiber may not be a practical solution to a patient who has advanced disease because daily fiber intake should increase by 450% to increase stool frequency by 50% [115].

Common laxatives that are used include bulk agents (methycellulose, bran), stool softeners (docusate sodium), saline laxatives (magnesium, hydroxide, magnesium citrate), osmotic laxatives (lactulose, sorbitol, polyethylene glycol), and enemas (tap water, sodium phosphate). Metoclopramide, a prokinetic, can be added to patients who may have gastrointestinal auto-nomic dysfunction; however, it is not a substitute for laxatives because it works primarily by binding to upper gastrointestinal receptors.

Because most patients who have advanced cancer also are taking high dosages of opioids, opioid antagonists, like naloxone, have been used clin-ically to reverse constipation that is secondary to opioids [116]. Its narrow therapeutic index and its potential for physical withdrawal symptoms limits its frequent use, however. Two drugs that are under investigation to treat this opioid-induced bowel dysfunction include methylnaltrexone [117] and alvimopan [118].

Summary

The key points of this article are

- Anorexia and cachexia are a major cause of cancer deaths. Several drugs are available to treat anorexia and cachexia.
- Dyspnea in cancer usually is caused by several factors. Treatment con-sists of reversing underlying causes, empiric bronchodilators, cortico-steroids—and in the terminally ill patients—opioids, benzodiazepines, and chlorpromazine.
- Delirium is associated with advanced cancer. Empiric treatment with neuroleptics while evaluating for reversible causes is a reasonable approach to management.
- Nausea and vomiting are caused by extra-abdominal factors (drugs, electrolyte abnormalities, central nervous system metastases) or intra-abdominal factors (gastroparesis, ileus, gastric outlet obstruction, bowel obstruction). The pattern of nausea and vomiting differs depending upon whether the cause is extra- or intra-abdominal. Reversible causes should be sought and empiric metoclopramide or haloperidol should be initiated.
- Fatigue may be caused by anemia, depression, endocrine abnormalities, or electrolyte disturbances that should be treated before using empiric methylphenidate.
- Constipation should be treated with laxatives and stool softeners. Both should start with the first opioid dose.

References

[1] Inui A. Cancer anorexia-cachexia syndrome: current issues in research and management. CA Cancer J Clin 2002;52(2):72–91.
[2] Bruera E. ABC of palliative care. Anorexia, cachexia, and nutrition. BMJ 1997;315(7117): 1219–22.
[3] Molassiotis A. Anorexia and weight loss in long-term survivors of haematological malignancies. J Clin Nurs 2003;12(6):925–7.
[4] Goldberg RM, Loprinzi CL. Cancer anorexia/cachexia. Cancer Treat Res 1999;100:31–41.

[5] Davis MP, Dreicer R, Walsh D, et al. Appetite and cancer-associated anorexia: a review. J Clin Oncol 2004;22(8):1510–7.

[6] Tisdale MJ. Cancer anorexia and cachexia. Nutrition 2001;17(5):438–42.

[7] Bosaeus I, Daneryd P, Svanberg E, et al. Dietary intake and resting energy expenditure in relation to weight loss in unselected cancer patients. Int J Cancer 2001;93(3):380–3.

[8] Costa G, Weathers AP. Cancer and the nutrition of the host. J Am Diet Assoc 1964;44: 15–7.

[9] Tisdale MJ. Metabolic abnormalities in cachexia and anorexia. Nutrition 2000;16(10): 1013–4.

[10] Holm E, Hagmuller E, Staedt U, et al. Substrate balances across colonic carcinomas in humans. Cancer Res 1995;55(6):1373–8.

[11] Holroyde CP, Gabuzda TG, Putnam RC, et al. Altered glucose metabolism in metastatic carcinoma. Cancer Res 1975;35(12):3710–4.

[12] Lundholm K, Edstrom S, Ekman L, et al. Metabolism in peripheral tissues in cancer patients. Cancer Treat Rep 1981;65(Suppl 5):79–83.

[13] Gibney E, Elia M, Jebb SA, et al. Total energy expenditure in patients with small-cell lung cancer: results of a validated study using the bicarbonate-urea method. Metabolism 1997; 46(12):1412–7.

[14] Warnold I, Lundholm K, Schersten T. Energy balance and body composition in cancer patients. Cancer Res 1978;38(6):1801–7.

[15] Lindmark L, Bennegard K, Eden E, et al. Resting energy expenditure in malnourished patients with and without cancer. Gastroenterology 1984;87(2):402–8.

[16] Hyltander A, Korner U, Lundholm KG. Evaluation of mechanisms behind elevated energy expenditure in cancer patients with solid tumours. Eur J Clin Invest 1993;23(1):46–52.

[17] Argiles JM, Moore-Carrasco R, Fuster G, et al. Cancer cachexia: the molecular mechanisms. Int J Biochem Cell Biol 2003;35(4):405–9.

[18] Argiles JM, Busquets S, Lopez-Soriano FJ. The role of uncoupling proteins in pathophysiological states. Biochem Biophys Res Commun 2002;293(4):1145–52.

[19] Sanders PM, Tisdale MJ. Effect of zinc-alpha(2)-glycoprotein (ZAG) on expression of uncoupling proteins in skeletal muscle and adipose tissue. Cancer Lett 2004;212(1): 71–81.

[20] Gercel-Taylor C, Doering DL, Kraemer FB, et al. Aberrations in normal systemic lipid metabolism in ovarian cancer patients. Gynecol Oncol 1996;60(1):35–41.

[21] Rofe AM, Bourgeois CS, Coyle P, et al. Altered insulin response to glucose in weight-losing cancer patients. Anticancer Res 1994;14(2B):647–50.

[22] Heber D, Byerley LO, Tchekmedyian NS. Hormonal and metabolic abnormalities in the malnourished cancer patient: effects on host-tumor interaction. JPEN J Parenter Enteral Nutr 1992;16(Suppl 6):60S–4S.

[23] Groundwater P, Beck SA, Barton C, et al. Alteration of serum and urinary lipolytic activity with weight loss in cachectic cancer patients. Br J Cancer 1990;62(5):816–21.

[24] Jeevanandam M, Horowitz GD, Lowry SF, et al. Cancer cachexia and the rate of whole body lipolysis in man. Metabolism 1986;35(4):304–10.

[25] Klein S, Wolfe RR. Whole-body lipolysis and triglyceride-fatty acid cycling in cachectic patients with esophageal cancer. J Clin Invest 1990;86(5):1403–8.

[26] Khan S, Tisdale MJ. Catabolism of adipose tissue by a tumour-produced lipid-mobilising factor. Int J Cancer 1999;80(3):444–7.

[27] Marshall MK, Doerrler W, Feingold KR, et al. Leukemia inhibitory factor induces changes in lipid metabolism in cultured adipocytes. Endocrinology 1994;135(1):141–7.

[28] Ishiko O, Yasui T, Hirai K, et al. Lipolytic activity of anemia-inducing substance from tumor-bearing rabbits. Nutr Cancer 1999;33(2):201–5.

[29] Ishiko O, Sumi T, Yoshida H, et al. Anemia-inducing substance is related to elimination of lipolytic hyperactivity by cyclic plasma perfusion in human cancer cachexia. Nutr Cancer 2000;37(2):169–72.

[30] Grunfeld C, Feingold KR. Regulation of lipid metabolism by cytokines during host defense. Nutrition 1996;12(Suppl 1):S24–6.

[31] Bing C, Bao Y, Jenkins J, et al. Zinc-alpha2-glycoprotein, a lipid mobilizing factor, is expressed in adipocytes and is up-regulated in mice with cancer cachexia. Proc Natl Acad Sci USA 2004;101(8):2500–5.

[32] Russell ST, Zimmerman TP, Domin BA, et al. Induction of lipolysis in vitro and loss of body fat in vivo by zinc-alpha2-glycoprotein. Biochim Biophys Acta 2004;1636(1):59–68.

[33] Attaix D, Combaret L, Tilignac T, et al. Adaptation of the ubiquitin-proteasome proteolytic pathway in cancer cachexia. Mol Biol Rep 1999;26(1–2):77–82.

[34] Hasselgren P-O, Wray C, Mammen J. Breakthroughs and views. Biochem Biophys Res Commun 2002;290:1–10.

[35] Giordano A, Calvani M, Petillo O, et al. Skeletal muscle metabolism in physiology and in cancer disease. J Cell Biochem 2003;90(1):170–86.

[36] Sarhill N, Mahmoud F, Walsh D, et al. Evaluation of nutritional status in advanced metastatic cancer. Support Care Cancer 2003;11(10):652–9.

[37] Ribaudo JM, Cella D, Hahn EA, et al. Re-validation and shortening of the Functional Assessment of Anorexia/Cachexia Therapy (FAACT) questionnaire. Qual Life Res 2000; 9(10):1137–46.

[38] Thoresen L, Fjeldstad I, Krogstad K, et al. Nutritional status of patients with advanced cancer: the value of using the subjective global assessment of nutritional status as a screening tool. Palliat Med 2002;16(1):33–42.

[39] Cella DF, VonRoenn J, Lloyd S, et al. The Bristol-Myers Anorexia/Cachexia Recovery Instrument (BACRI): a brief assessment of patients' subjective response to treatment for anorexia/cachexia. Qual Life Res 1995;4(3):221–31.

[40] Smith MR, Fuchs V, Anderson EJ, et al. Measurement of body fat by dual-energy X-ray absorptiometry and bioimpedance analysis in men with prostate cancer. Nutrition 2002; 18(7–8):574–7.

[41] Toso S, Piccoli A, Gusella M, et al. Altered tissue electric properties in lung cancer patients as detected by bioelectric impedance vector analysis. Nutrition 2000;16(2):120–4.

[42] Fredrix EW, Saris WH, Soeters PB, et al. Estimation of body composition by bioelectrical impedance in cancer patients. Eur J Clin Nutr 1990;44(10):749–52.

[43] Bozzetti F, Gavazzi C, Ferrari P, et al. Effect of total parenteral nutrition on the protein kinetics of patients with cancer cachexia. Tumori 2000;86(5):408–11.

[44] McCarthy DO. Rethinking nutritional support for persons with cancer cachexia. Biol Res Nurs 2003;5(1):3–17.

[45] Davis MP. New drugs for the anorexia-cachexia syndrome. Curr Oncol Rep 2002;4(3): 264–74.

[46] Argiles JM, Meijsing SH, Pallares-Trujillo J, et al. Cancer cachexia: a therapeutic approach. Med Res Rev 2001;21(1):83–101.

[47] De Conno F, Martini C, Zecca E, et al. Megestrol acetate for anorexia in patients with far-advanced cancer: a double-blind controlled clinical trial. Eur J Cancer 1998;34(11):1705–9.

[48] Jatoi A, Windschitl HE, Loprinzi CL, et al. Dronabinol versus megestrol acetate versus combination therapy for cancer-associated anorexia: a North Central Cancer Treatment Group study. J Clin Oncol 2002;20(2):567–73.

[49] Loprinzi CL, Schaid DJ, Dose AM, et al. Body-composition changes in patients who gain weight while receiving megestrol acetate. J Clin Oncol 1993;11(1):152–4.

[50] Barber MD, Ross JA, Fearon KC. Disordered metabolic response with cancer and its management. World J Surg 2000;24(6):681–9.

[51] Argiles JM, Moore-Carrasco R, Busquets S, et al. Catabolic mediators as targets for cancer cachexia. Drug Discov Today 2003;8(18):838–44.

[52] Burns CP, Halabi S, Clamon GH, et al. Phase I clinical study of fish oil fatty acid capsules for patients with cancer cachexia: cancer and leukemia group B study 9473. Clin Cancer Res 1999;5(12):3942–7.

[53] Barber MD, McMillan DC, Preston T, et al. Metabolic response to feeding in weight-losing pancreatic cancer patients and its modulation by a fish-oil-enriched nutritional supplement. Clin Sci (Lond) 2000;98(4):389–99.

[54] Wigmore SJ, Barber MD, Ross JA, et al. Effect of oral eicosapentaenoic acid on weight loss in patients with pancreatic cancer. Nutr Cancer 2000;36(2):177–84.

[55] Fainsinger RL, Waller A, Bercovici M, et al. A multicentre international study of sedation for uncontrolled symptoms in terminally ill patients. Palliat Med 2000;14(4):257–65.

[56] Bruera E, Schmitz B, Pither J, et al. The frequency and correlates of dyspnea in patients with advanced cancer. J Pain Symptom Manage 2000;19(5):357–62.

[57] Dudgeon DJ, Lertzman M. Dyspnea in the advanced cancer patient. J Pain Symptom Manage 1998;16(4):212–9.

[58] Dudgeon DJ, Lertzman M, Askew GR. Physiological changes and clinical correlations of dyspnea in cancer outpatients. J Pain Symptom Manage 2001;21(5):373–9.

[59] Gift AG. Validation of a vertical visual analogue scale as a measure of clinical dyspnea. Rehabil Nurs 1989;14(6):323–5.

[60] Gift AG, Narsavage G. Validity of the numeric rating scale as a measure of dyspnea. Am J Respir Crit Care Med 1998;7:200–4.

[61] Jennings AL, Davies AN, Higgins JP, et al. Opioids for the palliation of breathlessness in terminal illness. Cochrane Database of Systematic Reviews 2001(4):CD002066.

[62] Bruera E, Sala R, Spruyt O, et al. Nebulized versus subcutaneous morphine for the treatment of cancer dyspnea: a randomized, controlled trial. Support Care Cancer 2004; 12(6):405.

[63] Congleton J, Muers MF. The incidence of airflow obstruction in bronchial carcinoma, its relation to breathlessness, and response to bronchodilator therapy. Respir Med 1995;89(4): 291–6.

[64] Dudgeon DJ, Kristjanson L, Sloan JA, et al. Dyspnea in cancer patients: prevalence and associated factors. J Pain Symptom Manage 2001;21(2):95–102.

[65] Navigante AH, Castro MA, Cerchietti LC, et al. Oral morphine versus oral midazolam on dyspnea perception management. A prospective randomized study in ambulatory patients with cancer. Support Care Cancer 2004;12(6):420.

[66] Neill PA, Morton PB, Stark RD. Chlorpromazine—a specific effect on breathlessness? Br J Clin Pharmac 1985;19:793–7.

[67] Booth S, Kelly MJ, Cox NP, et al. Does oxygen help dyspnea in patients with cancer? Am J Respir Crit Care Med 1996;153(5):1515–8.

[68] Lawlor PG, Gagnon B, Mancini IL, et al. Occurrence, causes, and outcome of delirium in patients with advanced cancer: a prospective study. Arch Intern Med 2000;160(6): 786–94.

[69] Breitbart W, Gibson C, Tremblay A. The delirium experience: delirium recall and delirium-related distress in hospitalized patients with cancer, their spouses/caregivers, and their nurses. Psychosomatics 2002;43(3):183–94.

[70] Casarett DJ, Inouye SK. Diagnosis and management of delirium near the end of life. Ann Intern Med 2001;135(1):32–40.

[71] Trzepacz PT. Is there a final common neural pathway in delirium? Focus on acetylcholine and dopamine. Semin Clin Neuropsychiatry 2000;5(2):132–48.

[72] Johnson MH. Assessing confused patients. J Neurol Neurosurg Psychiatry 2001; 71(Suppl 1):i7–12.

[73] Lawlor PG. Delirium and dehydration: some fluid for thought? Support Care Cancer 2002; 10(6):445–54.

[74] Breitbart W, Tremblay A, Gibson C. An open trial of olanzapine for the treatment of delirium in hospitalized cancer patients. Psychosomatics 2002;43(3):175–82.

[75] Meagher DJ. Delirium: optimising management. BMJ 2001;322(7279):144–9.

[76] Schwartz TL, Masand PS. The role of atypical antipsychotics in the treatment of delirium. Psychosomatics 2002;43(3):171–4.

[77] Breitbart W, Marotta R, Platt MM, et al. A double-blind trial of haloperidol, chlorpro-
      mazine, and lorazepam in the treatment of delirium in hospitalized AIDS patients. Am J
      Psychiatry 1996;153(2):231–7.
[78] Cowan JD, Walsh D. Terminal sedation in palliative medicine—definition and review of the
      literature. Support Care Cancer 2001;9(6):403–7.
[79] Fainsinger R, Miller MJ, Bruera E, et al. Symptom control during the last week of life on
      a palliative care unit. J Palliat Care 1991;7(1):5–11.
[80] Curtis EB, Krech R, Walsh TD. Common symptoms in patients with advanced cancer.
      J Palliat Care 1991;7(2):25–9.
[81] Grond S, Zech D, Diefenbach C, et al. Prevalence and pattern of symptoms in patients with
      cancer pain: a prospective evaluation of 1635 cancer patients referred to a pain clinic. J Pain
      Symptom Manage 1994;9(6):372–82.
[82] Rhodes VA, McDaniel RW. Nausea, vomiting, and retching: complex problems in
      palliative care. CA Cancer J Clin 2001;51(4):232–48 [quiz 249–52].
[83] Davis MP, Walsh D. Treatment of nausea and vomiting in advanced cancer. Support Care
      Cancer 2000;8(6):444–52.
[84] Bruera E, Sweeney C. Chronic nausea and vomiting. In: Berger GM, Portenoy RK,
      Weissman DE, editors. Principles and practice of palliative care and supportive oncology.
      Philadelphia: Lippincott Williams & Wilkins; 2002. p. 57–60.
[85] Kinghorn S. Palliative care. Nausea and vomiting. Nurs Times 1997;93(33):57–60.
[86] Twycross R, Back I. Nausea and vomiting in advanced cancer. Eur J Palliat Care 1998;5:
      39–45.
[87] Bhana N, Foster RH, Olney R, et al. Olanzapine: an updated review of its use in the
      management of schizophrenia. Drugs 2001;61(1):111–61.
[88] Nelson KA, Walsh D. The use of cannabinoids in palliative medicine. Prog Palliative Care
      1998;6:160–3.
[89] Gandara DR, Harvey WH, Monaghan GG, et al. The delayed-emesis syndrome from
      cisplatin: phase III evaluation of ondansetron versus placebo. Semin Oncol 1992;
      19(4)(Suppl 10):67–71.
[90] Poli-Begelli S, Rodriguez-Pereira J, Carioes AD, et al for the Aprepitant Protocol 054
      Study Group. Addition of the neurokinin/receptor antagonist aprepitant to standard anti-
      emetic therapy improves control of chemotherapy-induced nausea and vomiting: results
      from a randomized, double-blind, placebo-controlled trial in Latin America. Cancer Lett
      2003;97:3090–8.
[91] Brooksbank MA, Game PA, Ashby MA. Palliative venting gastrostomy in malignant
      intestinal obstruction. Palliat Med 2002;16(6):520–6.
[92] Oishi H, Shindo H, Shirotani N, et al. The experience of improved quality of life at home for
      the long term, using percutaneous trans-esophageal gastro-tubing drainage for a cases with
      terminal stage cancer. J Tokyo Wom Med Univ 2001;71(3):188–92.
[93] Cella D, Davis K, Breitbart W, et al. Cancer-related fatigue: prevalence of proposed
      diagnostic criteria in a United States sample of cancer survivors. J Clin Oncol 2001;19(14):
      3385–91.
[94] Mock V, Piper B, Sabbatini P, et al. National comprehensive network fatigue practice
      guidelines. Oncology 2000;14(11A):151–61.
[95] Miaskowski CA, Portenoy RK. Fatigue. In: Berger AM, Portenoy RK, Weissman DE,
      editors. Principles and practice of palliative care and supportive oncology. Philadelphia:
      Lippincott Williams & Wilkins; 2002. p. 141–53.
[96] Nevenschwander H, Bruera E. Asthenia-cachexia. In: Bruera E, Higginson I, editors.
      Cachexia-anorexia in cancer patients. New York: Oxford University Press; 1996. p. 57–75.
[97] Krupp LB, LaRocca NG, Muir-Nash J, et al. The fatigue severity scale. Application to
      patients with multiple sclerosis and systemic lupus erythematosus. Arch Neurol 1989;
      46(10):1121–3.

[98] Rhoten D. Fatigue and the post-surgical patient. In: Concept clarification in nursing. Rockville (MD): ASPED; 1996. p. 277–300.

[99] Barnes EA, Bruera E. Fatigue in patients with advanced cancer: a review. Int J Gynecol Cancer 2002;12(5):424–8.

[100] Mendoza TR, Wang XS, Cleeland CS, et al. The rapid assessment of fatigue severity in cancer patients: use of the Brief Fatigue Inventory. Cancer 1999;85(5):1186–96.

[101] Piper B, Lindsey A, Dodd M, et al. The development of an instrument to measure the subjective dimension of fatigue. In: Funk S, Tornquist E, Champagne M, et al, editors. Key aspects of comfort management of pain fatigue and nausea. New York: Springer; 1989. p. 199–208.

[102] Chalder T, Berelowitz G, Pawlikowska T, et al. Development of a fatigue scale. J Psychosom Res 1993;37(2):147–53.

[103] Kaasa T, Loomis J, Gillis K, et al. The Edmonton Functional Assessment Tool: preliminary development and evaluation for use in palliative care. J Pain Symptom Manage 1997;13(1):10–9.

[104] Karnofsky DA, Burchenal JH. The clinical evaluation of chemotherapeutic agents in cancer. In: Macleod CM, editor. Evaluation of chemotherapeutic agents. New York: Columbia University Press; 1949. p. 191–205.

[105] Mock V. Fatigue management: evidence and guidelines for practice. Cancer 2001; 92(Suppl 6):1699–707.

[106] Dimeo FC. Effects of exercise on cancer-related fatigue. Cancer 2001;92(Suppl 6):1689–93.

[107] Sarhill N, Walsh D, Nelson KA, et al. Methylphenidate for fatigue in advanced cancer: a prospective open-label pilot study. Am J Hosp Palliat Care 2001;18(3):187–92.

[108] Rammwhan KW, Rosenberg JH, Lynn DJ, et al. Efficacy and safety of modafinil (provigil) for the treatment of fatigue in multiple sclerosis: a two center phase 2 study. J Neurol Neurosurg Psychiatry 2002;72:179–83.

[109] Bruera E, Roca E, Cedaro L, et al. Action of oral methylprednisolone in terminal cancer patients: a prospective randomized double-blind study. Cancer Treat Rep 1985;69(7–8): 751–4.

[110] Bruera E, Ernst S, Hagen N, et al. Effectiveness of megestrol acetate in patients with advanced cancer: a randomized, double-blind, crossover study. Cancer Prev Control 1998; 2(2):74–8.

[111] Levy M. Management of opioid-induced bowel dysfunction. J Nat Comp Cancer Network 2003;1(Suppl 3):522–6.

[112] Sykes N. The relationship between opioid use and laxative use in terminally ill cancer patients. Palliat Med 1998;12:375–82.

[113] Mancini I, Bruera E. Constipation in advanced cancer patients. Support Care Cancer 1998; 6:356–64.

[114] Kurz ASD. Opioid-induced bowel dysfunction. Drugs 2003;63(7):649–71.

[115] Sykes N. Constipation management in palliative care. Geriatric Med 1997;27:55–7.

[116] Sykes N. An investigation of the availability of oral naloxone to correct opioid-related constipation in patients with advanced cancer. Palliat Med 1996;10:135–44.

[117] Yuan CS, Foss JF, O'Connor M, et al. Methylnaltrexone for reversal of constipation due to chronic methadone use: a randomized controlled trial. JAMA 2000;283(3):367–72.

[118] Schmidt W. Alvimopan is a novel peripheral antagonist. Am J Surg 2001;182(Suppl 5A): 27S–38S.

ELSEVIER
SAUNDERS

SURGICAL
CLINICS OF
NORTH AMERICA

Surg Clin N Am 85 (2005) 257–272

Spiritual Issues in Surgical Palliative Care

Daniel B. Hinshaw, MD, FACS[a,b,*]

[a]Palliative Care Program and Surgical Service, Ann Arbor VA Medical Center,
2215 Fuller Road (112), Ann Arbor, MI 48105
[b]Department of Surgery, University of Michigan Medical School,
1500 East Medical Center Drive, Ann Arbor, MI 48109, USA

"For Americans, death is un-American, and an affront to every citizen's inalienable right to life, liberty and the pursuit of happiness" [1].

Every American will have the opportunity to experience this affront to the American way of life. This article represents an expansion and modification of themes that were presented elsewhere [2,3] and intends to find a common ground for understanding the spiritual issues that confront the dying and their surgeons in our highly diverse culture. Specifically, it (1) attempts to provide a working definition of spirituality in relation to religion; (2) explores the concept of a "good death" and whether current practice meets the expectations of the dying; (3) examines the nature of suffering and its relationship to spiritual distress; (4) identifies ways in which surgeons can alleviate spiritual distress; (5) examines the impact of grief on surgeons' care of their patients; and (6) explores the potential for healing in the terminally ill.

Spirituality

The major conclusion of a recent survey of 1200 adults in the United States was that "...the American people want to reclaim and reassert the spiritual dimension in dying" [4]. Spirituality has been described as "...a dimension of personhood defining the essence of humanity" [5]. It has been defined as "...that which allows a person to experience transcendent meaning in life. This is often expressed as a relationship with God, but it can

---

* Palliative Care Program and Surgical Service, Ann Arbor VA Medical Center, 2215 Fuller Road (112), Ann Arbor, MI 48105.
  E-mail address: hinshaw@umich.edu

also be about nature, art, music, family, or community—whatever beliefs and values give a person a sense of meaning and purpose in life" [6]. Also, "... spirituality focuses on a person's relationship to life itself. It is the person's innate drive to find meaning and purpose in his or her life and destiny. Some level of spiritual awareness graces the life of each person" [7]. Clearly, certain elements are common to these different definitions of spirituality. Many believe that it is the spiritual part of our nature that sets us apart from other creatures.

The search for purpose and meaning in life is perhaps the hallmark of spirituality, although many human beings may engage it only to varying extents. Ironically, it is sometimes only the threat of dissolution that is associated with a terminal diagnosis that awakens spiritual awareness within persons. The pertinence of the world's great religions to human spirituality has rested directly in how each addresses the questions of human suffering and death. Organized religion has provided a communal framework within which people may find a system of belief and action from which a sense of meaning and purpose can be derived.

Although religion has enriched spirituality in many ways, its relevance has been challenged by recent changes in popular culture. The highly individualistic and personalized approach to spiritual issues manifest in American culture from the colonial era to the present laid the foundation for much of the conflict and hostility toward organized religion that is seen in the United States today. The Gallup Index of Leading Religious Indicators has monitored the public perception of organized religion in America for more than 60 sixty years [8]. In January 2003, the Index demonstrated that public confidence in organized religion was at its lowest level in 6 decades. The Index includes eight different categories, five of which have remained fairly constant (first five listed) over the years and three that have varied considerably at times (last three listed) (Table 1).

Two of the three "variables" (the last two listed) demonstrated substantial change and reflected a decrease in public confidence in organized religion. Most of the change in these was attributed by poll analysts to the recent turmoil within the American branch of the Roman Catholic Church over alleged sexual misconduct among the clergy [8].

The issues with the American public's perception of organized religion go deeper, however, than an acute reaction to a clergy scandal, no matter how serious. In another Gallup poll (January, 2002), 50% of Americans described themselves as religious, 33% as "spiritual but not religious," 11% as neither religious nor spiritual, and 4% as religious and spiritual (2% were unaccounted for) [9]. Thus, one third of Americans—in keeping with the highly individualistic approach that many citizens have taken throughout the history of the United States—consciously eschew established religion in favor of a personally defined spirituality. Time will tell whether today's individual spiritual journey will become tomorrow's new sect or denomination. Certainly, American history suggests that we

Table 1
Public perception of organized religion in America

Leading religious indicators	% of positive respondents in 2001	% of positive respondents in 2002
Stated belief in God	95%	95%
Identified a religious preference	92%	90%
Membership in a faith community	56%	55%
Attended worship service in the last 7 days	41%	43%
Religion very important in one's life	58%	60%
Ability of religion to answer today's problems	62%	62%
Confidence in organized religion	60%	45%
Confidence in the clergy	64%	52%

await the birth of many new religious groups out of the current spiritual ferment.

These complexities raise the question: what are the implications for surgeons who may be concerned about how to address the spiritual needs of their terminally ill patients? At least for the foreseeable future, a large percentage of dying patients who experience spiritual distress may not respond well to approaches that are based purely in a traditional religious framework, even if the patient bears a specific religious label.

Looking for a "good death"

Considerable interest and effort have been concentrated on defining what it means to have a "good death." A recent focus group study examined the perceptions of dying patients, family members, and providers [10]. The study revealed six major components of a "good death": (1) effective pain and symptom management; (2) the ability to engage in clear decision making; (3) preparation for death; (4) a sense of completion; (5) continued ability to contribute to others; and (6) affirmation of the whole person. A particularly surprising finding to the investigators was the importance to dying patients of being able to contribute to others. At first, this may seem to be an unlikely priority for the dying; however, many seem to experience the great imperatives of human existence even more intensely when knowing that every moment counts.

Another striking feature of these results is that the last four components of a "good death" are primarily spiritual in nature. Even the first two often can have spiritual dimensions in context of the whole person. Sometimes, physical distress is a more socially and medically acceptable way to manifest deeper existential suffering.

In a large national survey (March–August, 1999) that complemented the aforementioned focus group study, the same investigators evaluated the perceptions of patients, family, physicians, and other providers (eg, nurses, social workers, chaplains, hospice volunteers) regarding the importance of 44 attributes of quality care at the end of life [11]. Twenty-six items were noted as important across all groups and included: effective pain and symptom management; preparation for death; achieving a sense of completion; being able to make decisions about treatment preferences; and being treated as a "whole person." Although there was excellent agreement across all of the groups with respect to these issues, disturbing and statistically significant $(P < .001)$ discrepancies were reported that involved several spiritual issues that were extremely important to dying patients, but were not so important to their physicians. These included: (1) being mentally aware; (2) being at peace with God; (3) not being a burden to one's family; (4) being able to help others; (5) being able to pray; (6) having funeral arrangements made; (7) not being a burden to society; and (8) feeling that one's life is complete.

Are physicians out of step with their dying patients? The great nineteenth century novelist, George Eliot, may have had real insight into this problem, which apparently also was present in nineteenth century English medical culture: "It is seldom a medical man has true religious views—there is too much pride of intellect" [12]. It is this apparent indifference to the spiritual aspect of care that often distinguishes physicians from the nurses, social workers, chaplains, and hospice volunteers that provide most palliative care services. In another qualitative study, 16 hospice patients from Seattle were interviewed regarding their attitudes about having spiritual discussions with their physicians [13]. Four major themes emerged to characterize physician behaviors that are important to these patients during such discussions (Box 1). Addressing these kinds of issues requires a relationship that is based on knowledge and trust. Modern surgical practice, with its short clinic visits and other time pressures, tends to militate against the formation of a surgeon–patient relationship that could engender such discussions.

Box 1. Dying patients' attitudes about spiritual discussions with their physicians

Treating the whole person—the dying do not want to be treated like statistics.

Treating with sensitivity—can the physician be discerning of the dying person's emotional state?

Favorable attitudes toward religious or spiritual discussions with doctors—patients viewed this as a real sign of a physician's interest in the patient as a person.

No preaching—spiritual/religious discussions should not be forced.

_____

Adapted from Hart A Jr, Kohlwes RJ, Deyo R, et al. Hospice patients' attitudes regarding spiritual discussion with their doctors. Am J Hosp Palliat Care 2003; 20(2):135–9.

The problems of inadequate physician support and communication in addressing the spiritual needs of dying patients may be intensified in the care of the dying child. In a retrospective analysis of the terminal care that was provided to 77 hospitalized dying children between the ages of 8 days and 16.8 years, only one case had clear documentation of a discussion with the dying child (a teenager) regarding the possibility of death [14]. Although it is possible that much younger (eg, school age) children may be able to have some real comprehension of the concept of death, this study suggests that most children who are dying in the hospital setting have limited opportunities to address their spiritual needs at the end of life, particularly if they are unaware that death is likely.

Another disturbing observation comes from a retrospective narrative analysis of medical records (eg, physician and nursing notes) in 200 adult deaths from a single institution [15]. It was observed that, "religious beliefs are documented in a paucity of abstractions, and sometimes reflect staff frustration with the unrealistic expectations of patient or family" [15]. This conclusion suggests that many busy providers are missing opportunities to address spiritual issues and may be misinterpreting the cues that are given by patients and their families. It also underscores the routinely inadequate documentation of religious/spiritual issues in the medical record.

An inherent conflict exists between the technique and technology of medicine and surgery, which are problem-focused and reductionist by nature, and the spiritual needs of the dying, which are rooted in mystery. "Death is the edge of a mystery, and turning our faces toward the problematic, through the persistent use of technology, at the hour of death keeps us from having to face mystery. Death is no problem to be solved; it resists any such formulation...By keeping our attention on end-of-life *problems*, we ignore the *mystery* of the end of life" [16]. Addressing the problems of the dying without caring for the person who is dying can miss opportunities to alleviate suffering. Attending to the whole person, including the spiritual aspect of each person, can contribute substantially to a "good death."

Suffering

At the heart of the spiritual distress of the dying is suffering. George Eliot observed that, "deep, unspeakable suffering may well be called a baptism, a regeneration, the initiation into a new state" [17]. It is critical for those who address the spiritual distress of the dying to fully understand the nature of suffering. Eric Cassel [18] defined suffering as "...the state of severe distress associated with events that threaten the intactness of the person." By its nature, "suffering is experienced by persons. Suffering occurs when an impending destruction of the person is perceived; it continues until the threat of disintegration has passed or until the integrity of the person can be restored in some other manner" [18]. The challenge at the end of life is to restore and maintain the integrity of the dying person in the face of a clear and ever present threat of disintegration. Suffering affects persons in all their complexity. "...Suffering can occur in relation to any aspect of the person, whether it is in the realm of social roles, group identification, the relation with self, body, or family, or the relation with a transpersonal, transcendent source of meaning" [18].

Another way to express the all-encompassing nature of suffering is the concept of "total pain" that was articulated by Dame Cicely Saunders [19], the founder of the modern hospice movement. She described four domains of pain that, in their totality, constitute "total pain" and suffering: physical pain (and other distressing physical symptoms); psychologic or emotional pain (eg, symptoms of anxiety and depression); social pain (eg, fear of separation from loved ones, broken relationships); and spiritual pain. Dr. Cassel also observed that if a caregiver does not recognize or diagnose suffering, s/he cannot relieve it [20].

Because suffering affects whole persons, the standard objective measures that are used to diagnose physical or psychologic diseases will not be helpful. Typically, suffering involves symptoms that threaten the patient's integrity as a person. The meaning of symptoms for an individual patient defines the nature of the suffering experienced; for example, if cancer-related pain is progressing, the fear of impending death can cause intense suffering. As a result, apparently simple symptoms may signify the deepest existential anguish of the patient who has a terminal illness. A unidimensional approach to symptom management—like providing opioid analgesics alone for the pain of progressing cancer—may not relieve the total pain of such a patient. Failure to recognize and treat suffering often is a reflection of caregivers' inability to focus on the person rather than the disease. Simply put, to make a diagnosis of suffering, one must be looking for it. Start by asking, "Are you suffering?" [20].

A case example may serve to illustrate the concept of total pain. "A" was a woman in her mid-50's who had advanced metastatic pancreatic cancer. Just before developing cancer, she was married happily for a second time after having been in an abusive relationship with her first husband. She was receiving high dosages of opioid analgesics with little relief for her intense abdominal and back pain. She could not understand why this was happening to her at a time when she finally had found a loving relationship. Her physical, psychologic, and spiritual distress were aggravated further by the social pain that she experienced in the presence of her grieving husband, who could not bear to let her go. Although she was being considered for a celiac plexus block as a more direct intervention to relieve her great distress, real relief of her pain could not come without a resolution of her social and spiritual distress that centered on her relationship with her husband. Ultimately, he needed to give her permission to die.

Total pain (suffering) affects the whole person. "...No man can be rendered pain free whilst he still wrestles with his faith. No man can come to terms with his God when every waking moment is taken up with pain or vomiting" [21].

Spiritual care of the dying

"...It is important to view spiritual care not as a compartmentalized feature of treatment but as an attitude that infuses the overall approach to wholeperson care, regardless of one's defined role in the care of the dying person" [5]. Because of the interdisciplinary team approach that is so central to palliative care, it is crucial that the attitude that underlies spiritual care become a collective property of the entire team. The first step in providing spiritual care is to take a spiritual history.

To identify better the spiritual needs of patients, Puchalski and Romer [6] developed a tool for taking a spiritual history. By taking a spiritual history, the surgeon endorses the importance of spirituality and gives the terminally ill patient permission to discuss spiritual issues. An acronym, FICA, is used to summarize key elements of the spiritual history and trigger questions that are useful in its discussion (Box 2).

When addressing the spiritual needs and concerns of terminally ill patients, there are several important principles for caregivers to keep in mind (Box 3).

For many patients and their surgeons, the need for control is a dominant force in their lives. Spiritual issues may lie dormant until the situation becomes desperate and beyond one's apparent control [22]. Facing a terminal illness is the quintessential threat to one's sense of control, and is the time when many spiritual concerns (long buried) may surface.

Many of the major spiritual concerns that Americans have about death were identified in the May 1997 Gallup survey (Table 2) [4]. Many dying

---

Box 2. Taking a spiritual history

Faith—Do you consider yourself religious or spiritual? Do you have a faith? (If there is a negative response to these questions—What gives meaning to your life?)
Importance—Is it important (or how important is it) in your life?
Community—Are you part of a spiritual (or faith) community?
Address—How can your health care providers address—and respect—these issues in your care?

Adapted from Puchalski C, Romer L. Taking a spiritual history allows physicians to understand patients more fully. J Palliat Med 2000;3:131.

Box 3. Principles of spiritual care

Spirituality is an essential component of each person.
Spirituality is an ongoing issue—readdress it over time.
Demonstrate consistent respect for a patient's values, autonomy,
    and vulnerability. Do not impose your beliefs on a vulnerable
    patient.
Refer frequently to chaplains and spiritual directors with the
    consent and desire of the patient.
Know yourself! "...You can't address a patient's spirituality until
    you address your own."

Adapted from Puchalski C, Romer L. J Palliat Med 2000;3:129–37.

---

patients will be unable to verbalize their spiritual anguish; consequently, surgeons will need to be alert to signs of spiritual distress. Some of these signs include physical distress (eg, pain) that is unresponsive to standard therapies, acting out or refusal to cooperate (the "bad" patient), emotional withdrawal, and fears of loss of control or increasing dependence. Denial is defense mechanism that patients who have advanced illnesses frequently use as they struggle with the distressing side effects and poor odds that are associated with "last ditch" therapies. Denial can deepen spiritual distress by preventing its identification and recognition by the dying patient. Typically, clinicians are wary of confronting a patient's system of denial. "Clinicians agree that denial generally should not be challenged when a patient is in the midst of a crisis because doing so risks undermining the patient's psychological equilibrium" [23]. How often have we missed an opportunity to uncover and address spiritual distress when we follow this precept? Death is the last crisis that each person must face. It also is the last opportunity for spiritual growth.

   In addressing the spiritual distress of the dying, one investigator suggested that it is important to distinguish between religious and spiritual

Table 2
Major spiritual concerns of Americans about death

Concern	Percentage of positive respondents
Not being forgiven by God	56%
Not being reconciled with others	56%
Dying while being cut off or removed from God or a higher power	51%
Not being forgiven by someone for a past offense	49%
Not having a blessing from a family member or clergy member	39%
The nature of the experience after death	39%

pain. Religious pain has been defined as "...a condition in which a patient is feeling guilty over the violation of the moral codes and values of his or her religious tradition," whereas, "patients in spiritual pain are those who have concluded, through their own self judgments, that there is something wrong with them at their core" [24]. Religious faith at the end of life can be a two-edged sword. If faith has been integrated consistently throughout the person's life and actions, it can be a great support when the crisis of dying raises a host of spiritual issues; however, if a person's life and behavior has not been well-integrated or consistent with one's professed faith, this religious "dissonance" can only compound, or even create, spiritual distress.

It also is important to recognize the intersection of culture and spirituality in care at the end of life [25]. The Western emphasis on individual autonomy can create conflicts in the care of patients with cultural and religious traditions that differ from the dominant culture. Decision-making and communication in some cultures (eg, Mediterranean) may be more family-based or delegated to another family member. Perceived and real inequities in health care access or historical quality of care may influence a whole subculture's approach to various issues (eg, frequent reluctance of African Americans to request "do not resuscitate orders" and lower enrollment in hospice). Some cultures are reticent to discuss death directly (eg, Japanese, Native Americans). The Western "right to know" can be in direct conflict with the perceived power of the spoken word; what is not said explicitly may not become reality. Seeking support for dying loved ones from agencies that are outside of the family (eg, hospice) may be viewed in some cultures (eg, Hispanic) as a failure to fulfill one's responsibility. Although many surgeons are familiar with the cultural nuances of their communities, interdisciplinary support can be important when addressing particular spiritual challenges in diverse practices. Community-based clergy and social workers are among the resources that can be helpful in these situations.

Hospice is facing new challenges as American culture continues to evolve. A cherished core value of hospice philosophy has been the assumption that most people want to die at home. Although this may have been an easier sell in the 1970s when the modern hospice movement began in America, profound changes in the culture (eg, double-income families, an increasingly mobile and rootless society) have militated against this ideal. Seventy-five percent of people die in an institutional setting; in the large national survey that was quoted earlier [11], dying at home was not identified as the highest priority. Nonetheless, "home" is an important therapeutic concept. "Within the home environment, the dying person is among familiar surroundings and can be more at ease yielding to the spiritual journey of searching for meaning and purpose in his or her life" [26]. The challenge is to create an experience of "home" for that majority who will die in an institution.

The following case example illustrates the potential power of a patient's spirituality in the relief of suffering. "C" was a woman in her early 70s who presented with a locally advanced unresectable colon cancer that had replaced the lower half of her abdominal wall with a large, malodorous, fungating mass. The nursing staff had noted that she rarely required pain medications and often was found in deep, meditative prayer. When asked about how she was coping with her affliction, her response without hesitation was to quote the tenth verse of Psalm 46: "Be still, and know that I am God!".

The surgeon and grief

The emotional burden that is carried by each person who cares for critically ill and dying patients can be overwhelming at times and may limit one's ability to interact effectively in the healing encounter. Surgeons may be particularly vulnerable to the effects of caregiver grief; the relationships that they form with their patients often are predicated on a multiplicity of factors that tie them on an emotional level closely to their patients' outcomes. Factors that are unique to the surgeon–patient relationship include: (1) the often "high-stakes" nature of surgical interventions where success can mean cure or significant improvement in quality of life but failure may mean death or significant long-term suffering and disability for the patient; (2) the intimate nature of many surgical interventions in which the patient's "privacy" (ie, physical person) is invaded so directly; (3) the reciprocal effect that this surgical "intimacy" has on the surgeon—often producing great joy ("the surgeon's rush") with every success but a joy that often is haunted by the dread that the operation or its aftermath may not go well; and (4) the longstanding tradition within medicine, especially surgery, of placing great value on emotional detachment and distancing from one's patients. Perhaps in no other area of medical specialization does the physician place his/her ego in a more vulnerable position than in the practice of surgery. The emotional bond that forms between surgeon and patient often is un-recognized at a conscious level by the surgeon. It may be limited with the quick encounter of an uncomplicated outpatient procedure; however, it tends to grow in intensity in relation to the complexity of the procedure, its inherent risks, the duration of inpatient care, any complications that occur, and how the outcome reflects the surgeon's sense of self worth.

Observations that were published regarding the grieving process among the bereaved also may be pertinent to recognizing the grief that surgeons may experience in their practice. Bereavement has been defined as the experience of loss by death of a person to whom one is attached; mourning has been defined as the process of adapting to such a loss; and grief has been defined as the thoughts, feelings, and behaviors that one experiences after the loss [27]. A fundamental question with respect to surgeons and grief would seem to be: Is it not true that surgeons often become emo-tionally attached to their patients, although perhaps being unaware of this attachment, and in their losses frequently meet the definition of bereavement above? Are there risks associated with not recognizing one's grief? Various forms of complicated or abnormal grief have been identified [27]. Of the different forms of complicated grief, surgeons may be particularly vulnerable to experiencing delayed and masked grief. The following case example illustrates the effect of delayed grief in the life of a surgeon. A busy Midwestern surgeon is unable to be present for much of the gradual decline and death of his elderly mother in California secondary to multiple debilitating chronic illnesses. Although he is present for her funeral and the brief family gathering afterward, he plunges back into the intense clinical routine of his work immediately after returning home. A month later, he is informed by an inpatient hospice of the death from recurrent disease of one of his patients whom he had been following closely for nearly 3 years after a Whipple procedure for pancreatic adenocarcinoma. At this moment he is struck with an overwhelming wave of grief for this patient and his mother.

Much interest has been focused recently on physician (including surgeon) burnout [28,29]. Much of the fatigue, emotional exhaustion, and uncertainty about the meaning and value of one's work that is experienced during burnout, may, in truth, be a reflection of masked grief. Because surgeons have been trained not to show emotion or acknowledge their grief, they may not have any healthy options available to them for addressing their own distress from loss within their personal and professional lives. The lack of recognition of the problem may be coupled with a sense of shame when a surgeon encounters the frightening experience of powerful emotions that are difficult to control.

The surgeon's grief may be complicated further by the events that surround the patient's death. Unresolved conflicts at the time of a patient's death with other members of the health care team or with the patient's family can become an unhealthy drain of much emotional energy for the surgeon. Discussions in morbidity and mortality conferences often may exacerbate the problem; too often the focus becomes an effort to provide a rationalization and justification for actions taken, rather than an opportunity to express regret for the loss of the patient. Likewise, the grief of a surgeon after the loss of a patient following a long and complicated postoperative course is compounded when the survivors make a decision to address their grief in the form of a tort claim. Such a turn of events transforms the focus from shared loss to an adversarial relationship in which little healing is likely to occur.

Experience from hospice and palliative care has demonstrated a potential alternative approach to addressing the surgeon's grief. For grief to resolve, real mourning must occur. Some of the key elements in the process of mourning include accepting and experiencing the pain and reality of the loss, and remembering the deceased while moving forward with one's life [27]. Making time for reflection on the spiritual aspects of one's clinical work is a luxury that seldom is available to busy surgeons. With the advent of hospital-based palliative care programs, however, many more hospitals have regularly scheduled memorial services for patients who died within their health care system. A common practice at such memorial services is an oral recitation of the names of those patients who are being remembered. The experience of hearing the name of one's patient in such a context can bring back many powerful memories (good and bad) and reorient them in the context of an overt recognition of the patient's deceased condition. Having this experience some months (usually at least 6 months) after the patient's death with the patient's family, friends, and other hospital staff invited to participate creates a venue that is more conducive for healing of relationships and any remaining painful memories.

The potential for healing in death

"In my end is my beginning." With this last sentence of the second of his *Four Quartets (East Coker)*, TS Eliot [30] expresses all of the potential for renewal of hope and discovery of meaning that the terminally ill seek as they face death. The word "end" has two meanings that are expressed in ancient Greek as two different words, both of which are directly relevant to the spiritual struggle of the dying—end as a "state of completion or maturity" ("telos") and end as "last" in time ("eschatos") [31]. It is the discovery and experience of these two qualities of the end—balancing a full awareness of having arrived at the last stage of one's life with a sense of the opportunity for completion and full maturation—that can transform one's end into a beginning. For example, one patient who was dying slowly after struggling for several years with metastatic breast cancer was able to observe that she had not really begun to live until she faced her own mortality. Morrie Schwartz was the subject of a best-selling book—entitled *Tuesdays with Morrie*, about his dying from amyotrophic lateral sclerosis. He stated this principle succinctly, "When you learn how to die, you learn how to live" [32].

Paradoxically, the threat of loss and separation that are associated with death and anticipated bereavement can be powerful opportunities for spiritual growth and healing for the dying and for those who survive. Bereavement is a crisis that can trigger spiritual change if: (1) the situation creates a psychologic dysequilibrium that resists easy stabilization; (2) there is time for reflection; and (3) the person's life is forever colored by the experience [33]. Thus, real potential for healing in death exists not only for the dying person, but also for the family and loved ones who will remain, and even for the caregivers. This potential for healing begins with a redefinition of hope. Hope has been defined in the context of terminal illness as the "positive expectation for meaning attached to life events" [34]. "Hope lies in *meaning* that is attached to life, not in events themselves." Ultimately, "...as long as there is meaning, there is hope." It is a loss of meaning and a loss of hope that often underlie requests for physician-assisted suicide.

Several factors are crucial to helping dying patients as they redefine hope [34]. Patients need to know that they are dying. This understanding is critical before a successful transition from the role of being sick to that of dying can occur. Hospice referral and interdisciplinary support can facilitate this transition by creating a new identity and point of reference for the dying patient. Hope can be redefined in terms that are appropriate to the new circumstances. The clear and unambiguous commitment of caregivers to the dying patient generates hope. This commitment should include strong reassurance that the dying person will not be abandoned, that pain and other distressing symptoms will be controlled, that the dying person will be remembered, and that reconciliation and forgiveness can occur.

One tool that has been used in hospice care to help patients find meaning at the end of life is the preparation of a patient's biography [35]. Volunteer "biographers" first record the dying person's autobiography on tape and then prepare a written transcript, which is bound, for the patient to pass on to loved ones. "Life review enables a person to identify what has been accomplished or created, and what will be left behind as a result...a sense of meaning may be captured in the recognition of the uniqueness of the individual" [35].

Sometimes, medications, procedures, and even words are not enough. It requires great self-discipline, but just being present may be exactly what is needed—not only for the dying patient but also for the surgeon. "Listening is one of the greatest spiritual gifts a chaplain can give a suffering patient" [36]. This principle is not only applicable to chaplains, but to all caregivers. Comforting presence also can be provided in the context of various forms of complementary and alternative therapies (eg, massage, music, art therapy). As an example, for music therapy to be helpful, knowing the patient's musical "history" is important. Music (and other complementary therapies) sometimes can serve as the catalyst for release (emotional and spiritual) at the end of life [37].

Reconciliation also is central to the work of the dying. It extends the healing that they can experience beyond themselves to others. "Reconciliation is the most crucial thing for the dying irrespective of whether or not the person is religious or secular. Even as their bodies are disintegrating they are becoming whole" [38]. Ira Byock described the work of reconciliation for the dying and those they love as occurring in five steps: "Forgive me; I forgive you; Thank you; I love you; and Good-bye" [34].

A case example may help to illustrate how family healing and reconciliation can occur in the midst of intense suffering. "S" was a women in her late 50s who had widely metastatic lung cancer with multiple, extremely painful cutaneous and soft tissue metastases. She had a deep religious faith and was able to say that her affliction had been a blessing by bringing her children back to faith and confirming a religious vocation for her husband.

Changes in a dying person's dream life can be deeply affecting, and frequently signal the transition to active dying. Vivid, and often symbolic, dreams may occur (eg, taking a journey, finishing a building project) in which the dying person is uncertain of being awake or asleep. Also, the dying person may be found speaking to unseen presences, often deceased loved ones. Although these experiences may be comforting to the dying individual, they may be perplexing to loved ones or dismissed (and treated) as delirium by physicians; however, such events may represent another level of reconciliation that occurs within the dying person—reconciliation with the process of dying. These experiences before the onset of active dying should not be confused with the so-called "near death experience," which may occur in conjunction with a cardiac arrest [39]. In the near death experience, the individual who survives cardiac arrest typically describes an "out of body" experience which may include seeing one's own body and seeing and hearing the health care team discussing one's death, while, often at the same time, being drawn toward a light. The experience often ends in the distressing recognition of the necessity to return to bodily existence. Both types of experience have a transformative quality. The vivid, symbolic dreams and encounters with deceased loved ones help to prepare the dying person for the final stages of the dying process. The near death experience may awaken a dormant spirituality that could lead to real religious commitment and a source of peace regarding one's mortality.

How can surgeons experience healing through the death of their patients? Several critical opportunities for personal growth are presented to those who witness, attempt to alleviate, and experience the suffering of the dying. Observing and really seeing the death of a terminally ill patient can break down one's own denial of death. The grace that so many patients exhibit as they die can overcome the fear of death and sense of failure in the face of death that so many surgeons experience. Finally, and perhaps most important, is the opportunity to find and fully experience empathy—empathy for the dying patient, empathy for the family and loved ones, and empathy for the other members of the team of caregivers who also have suffered with the patient and family.

There are barriers to empathy. To have pain is "to have certainty." The patient has this certainty; the surgeon does not. Surgeons, in developing empathy, must overcome their tendency to doubt the patient. They should listen to their patient's complaints of pain (their suffering) "not to explain but to understand, not to diagnose but to witness and help" [40]. Sometimes, patients are not particularly likeable; they may be abusive and threatening to the surgeon. Finding a common history or shared experience can serve as a bridge in developing a relationship of caring for the "difficult" patient [41].

Jerome, the late fourth-century scholar and translator of the Scriptures into Latin, may have described best the common bond in our humanity that draws forth empathy in the face of suffering. "He whom we look down upon, whom we cannot bear to see, the very sight of whom causes us to vomit, is the same as we, formed with us from the selfsame clay, compacted of the same elements. Wherever he suffers we also can suffer" [42]. Empathy can and should be the end and the beginning for all who care for the dying.

Summary

The key points of this article are:

- Spirituality gives meaning and purpose to life. Spiritual issues that may lie dormant for many years often surface at the end of life. Not all people are religious, but all are spiritual.
- Suffering affects the whole person and often is connected to the meaning that a patient associates with a symptom or symptoms.
- Spiritual history validates the importance of a patient's spirituality and gives permission to the patient for future discussion/questions.
- Spiritual care is the job of all members of the interdisciplinary team (including surgeons), not just chaplains. It is critical to be open to spiritual discussions/issues as they arise while seeking the assistance of professional pastoral care staff where appropriate.
- Redefining hope: hospice can help the dying patient to redefine hope in terms of realistic goals—from a hope for cure to a hope for good symptom relief.
- Reconciliation is the work of the dying.
- Empathy is the opportunity for those who care for the dying.

References

[1] Toynbee A, Mant A, Smart N, et al. Changing attitudes towards death in the Western world. In: Toynbee A, et al, editor. Man's concern with death. New York: McGraw Hill; 1968. p. 131–280.

[2] Hinshaw DB. The spiritual needs of the dying patient. J Am Coll Surg 2002;195(4):565–9.

[3] Hinshaw DB. Spiritual issues at the end of life. Clin Fam Pract 2004;6(2):423–40.

[4] The George H Gallup International Institute. Spiritual beliefs and the dying process, a report of a national survey conducted for the Nathan Cummings Foundation and Fetzer Institute. Princeton (NJ): The George H Gallup International Institute; 1997.

[5] Kaut KP. Religion, spirituality, and existentialism near the end of life—implications for assessment and application. Am Behav Scientist 2002;46:220–34.

[6] Puchalski C, Romer AL. Taking a spiritual history allows clinicians to understand patients more fully. J Palliat Med 2000;3:129–37.

[7] O'Connell LJ. Changing the culture of dying. A new awakening of spirituality in America heightens sensitivity to needs of dying persons. Health Prog 1996;77:16–20.

[8] Gallup G Jr. Gallup Index of Leading Religious Indicators. Gallup poll Tuesday briefing, January 7, 2003. Available at: http://www.gallup.com. Accessed January 7, 2003.

[9] Gallup GH Jr. Americans' spiritual searches turn inward. Gallup poll Tuesday briefing, February 11, 2003. Available at http://www.gallup.com. Accessed February 11, 2003.

[10] Steinhauser KE, Clipp EC, McNeilly M, et al. In search of a good death: observations of patients, families, and providers. Ann Intern Med 2000;132:825–32.

[11] Steinhauser KE, Christakis NA, Clipp EC, et al. Factors considered important at the end of life by patients, family, physicians, and other care providers. JAMA 2000;284: 2476–82.

[12] Enck RE. Connecting the medical and spiritual models in patients nearing death. Am J Hosp Palliat Care 2003;20(2):88–92.

[13] Hart A Jr, Kohlwes RJ, Deyo R, et al. Hospice patients' attitudes regarding spiritual discussions with their doctors. Am J Hosp Palliat Care 2003;20(2):135–9.

[14] McCallum DE, Byrne P, Bruera E. How children die in hospital. J Pain Symptom Manage 2000;20:417–23.

[15] Fins JJ, Schwager Guest R, Acres CA. Gaining insight into the care of hospitalized dying patients: an interpretive narrative analysis. J Pain Symptom Manage 2000;20:399–407.

[16] Bevins M, Cole T. Ethics and spirituality: strangers at the end of life? In: Lawton MP, editor. Annual review of gerontology and geriatrics, focus on the end of life: scientific and social issues. New York: Springer Publishing Co; 2000. p. 20–7.

[17] Steensma DP. Why me? Journal of Clinical Oncology 2003;21(9)(Suppl):64s–6s.

[18] Cassel EJ. The nature of suffering and the goals of medicine. New Engl J Med 1982;306: 639–45.

[19] Saunders C, Sykes N. The management of terminal malignant disease. 3rd edition. London: Edward Arnold; 1993.

[20] Cassel EJ. Diagnosing suffering: a perspective. Ann Intern Med 1999;131:531–4.

[21] Doyle D, Hanks G, MacDonald N. Oxford textbook of palliative medicine. 2nd edition. New York: Oxford University Press; 1998.

[22] Friedemann M-L, Mouch J, Racey T. Nursing the spirit: the framework of systemic organization. J Adv Nurs 2002;39(4):325–32.

[23] Block SD. Psychological considerations, growth, and transcendence at the end of life. The art of the possible. JAMA 2001;285:2898–905.

[24] Satterly L. Guilt, shame, and religious and spiritual pain. Holist Nurs Pract 2001;15(2): 30–9.

[25] Thomas ND. The importance of culture throughout all of life and beyond. Holist Nurs Pract 2001;15(2):40–6.

[26] Vassallo BM. The spiritual aspects of dying at home. Holist Nurs Pract 2001;15(2): 17–29.

[27] Worden JW. Bereavement care. In: Berger AM, Portenoy RK, Weissman DE, editors. Principles and practice of palliative care and supportive oncology. 2nd edition. Philadelphia: Lippincott Williams and Wilkins; 2002. p. 813–8.

[28] Ramirez AJ, Graham J, Richards MA, et al. Burnout and psychiatric disorder among cancer clinicians. Br J Cancer 1995;71(6):1263–9.

[29] Campbell DA Jr, Sonnad SS, Eckhauser FE, et al. Burnout among American surgeons. Surgery 2001;130(4):696–705.

[30] Eliot TS. Four quartets. New York: Harcourt Brace Jovanovich; 1971.

[31] Liddell HG, Scott R. A Greek–English lexicon. London: Oxford University Press; 1973.

[32] Albom M. Tuesdays with Morrie, an old man, a young man and life's greatest lesson. New York: Doubleday; 1997.

[33] Balk DE. Bereavement and spiritual change. Death Stud 1999;23:485–93.

[34] Parker-Oliver D. Redefining hope for the terminally ill. Am J Hospice Palliat Care 2002;19: 115–20.

[35] Lichter I, Mooney J, Boyd M. Biography as therapy. Palliat Med 1993;7:133–7.

[36] Burns S. The spirituality of dying. Pastoral care's holistic approach is crucial in hospice. Health Prog 1991;72:48–54.

[37] Krout RE. Music therapy with imminently dying hospice patients and their families: facilitating release near the time of death. Am J Hospice Palliat Care 2003;20(2):129–34.

[38] Guroian V. Life's living toward dying, a theological and medical-ethical study. Grand Rapids (MI): William B Eerdmans Publishing Co; 1996.

[39] Nelson HR. The near death experience: observations and reflections from a retired chaplain. J Pastor Care 2000;54(2):159–66.

[40] Schweizer H. To give suffering a language. Lit Med 1995;14:210–21.

[41] Liaschenko J. Making a bridge: the moral work with patients we do not like. J Palliat Care 1994;10:83–9.

[42] Risse GB. Mending bodies, saving souls: a history of hospitals. Oxford (UK): Oxford University Press; 1999.

ELSEVIER
SAUNDERS

Surg Clin N Am 85 (2005) 273–286

SURGICAL
CLINICS OF
NORTH AMERICA

Ethical Issues in Surgical Palliative Care: Am I Killing the Patient by "Letting Him Go"?

Timothy M. Pawlik, MD, MPH*,
Steven A. Curley, MD

*Department of Surgical Oncology, The University of Texas M. D. Anderson Cancer Center,
Unit 444, P.O. Box 301402, 1515 Holcombe Boulevard, Houston, TX 77030, USA*

Decision-making around terminal care always has been difficult. The ability of medicine to prolong biologic life through the use of technology and pharmacology, however, has complicated further the role of physicians in treating the critically or terminally ill. In some sense, the benefits of medical advances have introduced a new set of burdens. Whereas disease processes, such as cardiopulmonary failure and sepsis, were the harbingers of a speedy death in the past, we often now have the capacity to sustain biologic life and prevent a "gentle, peaceful, and natural" death. Instead, the dying process today occurs almost invariably in highly mechanized and technology-driven environments, such as the ICU. Furthermore, decisions about forgoing life-sustaining therapies and implementing palliative care are becoming more prevalent in today's ICUs [1,2]. Surveys have shown that between 40% and 70% of ICU deaths follow the decision to forgo cardiopulmonary resuscitation or other forms of life-sustaining therapies [3,4]. Given this, it is critically important that surgeons are aware of the ethical considerations that contribute to clinical decision-making at the end of life.

The practice of ethics

One of the fundamental challenges for bioethics is to help delineate the process by which one terminates treatment for patients who are critically or terminally ill. Given the lack of professional practice standards and the nuanced issues that are involved in deliberations around death and dying,

* Corresponding author.
E-mail address: tmpawlik@mdanderson.org (T.M. Pawlik).

surgeons often are ill-equipped to confront decisions to stop life-sustaining therapies. In these circumstances, ethics can act as a guide to provide surgeons with concrete analytic tools to help frame end-of-life dilemmas. Surgical ethics does this by asking "what should guide the conduct of surgeons?" and "what ought the character of the surgeon be?".

Principles of moral reasoning

Moral reasoning in the medical context can be drawn from a wide range of ethical theories and perspectives. Some approaches to ethics are normative (ie, they establish standards of right or good action), whereas other approaches focus on virtue or character (ie, they concentrate more on the persons who are making the ethical decisions as compared with the decision itself) or emphasize middle-level ethical principles (ie, they center on key moral duties or principles, instead of pursuing difficult foundational issues). It is this last mode of moral reasoning, the principled approach, that has received the most attention in medical ethics.

Principles are general guides that leave room for judgment in specific cases and provide substantive guidance for the development of more detailed rules. The four clusters of principles as proposed by Beauchamp and Childress [5] are (1) respect for autonomy, (2) nonmaleficence, (3) beneficence, and (4) justice (Table 1). Each principle highlights an overarching ethical value. For example, autonomy bids us to respect the capacity of individuals to choose their own destiny, whereas justice calls us to act fairly and to distribute burdens and benefits in an equitable fashion. When faced with ethical dilemmas that concern end-of-life issues, surgeons can use these four principles to help guide their decisions. The process of applying and balancing the four clusters of moral principles, however, can be problematic and cannot be dictated rigidly by a predetermined formula. No one principle enjoys automatic supremacy over the others, rather ethical deliberations require a weighing and balancing of the various principles against one another in each concrete situation. Thus, although principles offer an important departure point and may help to structure ethical decision-making, an overreliance on them can be simplistic, and ultimately, detrimental. It often is difficult to determine which principle pertains to any given situation and how the principle should be applied. For example, autonomy may imply that a patient's wish to withdraw ventilator support be honored, whereas nonmaleficence could be argued to suggest that such a move would harm the patient by expediting his or her death. In these types of cases, the individual surgeon's character shapes how he or she attempts to balance conflicting principles.

Character as moral guide

Issues of character are important in how a physician participates in end-of-life decision-making [6]. What we endeavor to do morally is "not in itself determined by the rules (or principles) that we adhere to or how we respond

Table 1
Principles of biomedical ethics [5]

Principle	Ethical imperative
Autonomy	Respect the capacity of individuals to make their own choices and act accordingly
Nonmaleficence	Do no harm; one ought not to inflict pain or suffering
Beneficence	Foster the interests and happiness of other persons and society; prevent or treat pain and suffering
Justice	Act fairly; resolve dilemmas using fair and proportional means; distribute benefits and harms equitably

to one particular situation, but what we have become through our past history, by our character" [7]. The meaning of character denotes a set of specifiable traits and dispositions on the part of the surgeon. Character is the "qualification of our self-agency, formed by our having certain intentions (and beliefs) rather than others" [7]. Integrity of character is identified with consistency and moral strength. Character provides a link with intentions and forms part of the background of our judgments. A rightly-formed character cares about a morally appropriate response to a situation. When informed by character, a surgeon is not simply following rules of obligation or action-guides; rather, the surgeon is striving to do what is morally right out of a sense of motivation and desire to perform right actions. Character gives us orientation and direction to our lives and provides us with a foundation upon which to deal with our ethical struggles. An ethics of character challenges surgeons to examine the ethical situation and themselves as ethical decision-makers. Ethical principles that are informed by character can assist surgeons who find themselves confronted by ambiguity and uncertainty around end-of-life decision-making.

Decisional capacity: autonomous decision-making

Autonomy

The word autonomy, derived from the Greek *autos* ("self") and *nomos* ("rule") first was used to refer to the self-rule of the Hellenic city-states [5]. Autonomy has since acquired the meanings of privacy, individual choice, freedom of will, and the right to self-determination. Ethics and law place a premium on patient autonomy, defined as the right to be a fully informed participant in all aspects of medical decision-making and the right to refuse unwanted, even recommended, life-saving medical care. The principle of autonomy recognizes that each patient has a fundamental right to control his or her body and to be protected from unwanted intrusions. Autonomy or self-determination is independently valuable—we value it in itself as recognition of our "self" by an "other." The judicial system similarly has acknowledged the importance of self-determination. In numerous legal cases, the courts consistently have reaffirmed that the refusal of treatment by a competent individual must be respected. Given this, when a decision to shift from life-sustaining therapies to palliative care is begun, the patient always should be involved directly in all discussions and decision-making processes. Open discussions with the patient help to decipher his or her exact wishes around end-of-life choices and allow him or her to maintain dignity as a moral autonomous agent. If the patient is able to participate in decision-making actively, his or her contemporary wishes always should take precedence over any wish that was expressed in a previously written advanced directive.

Advance directives

Sixty to 70% of seriously ill patients are unable to speak for themselves when decisions to limit treatment are considered [8,9]. In addition, only 10% to 20% of patients have completed advance directives [10]; these usually only apply to patients who clearly are terminally ill or permanently unconscious, categories that often are inapplicable to many patients in the ICU [11]. Physicians, therefore, need to be aware of the various approaches to deal with incompetent patients' wishes at the end of life.

The term "living will" was described first in 1969 by Luis Kutner as a document in which a competent adult set forth directions regarding medial treatment in the event that he or she become incapacitated in the future [10]. With an advance directive, a patient who currently is incompetent can be treated or not treated according to his or her own previously expressed wishes. Advance directives are helpful in that they can identify preemptively certain desires and values that a patient may have around specific issues of death and dying (eg, long-term ventilator management, wish to avoid persistent vegetative state). Rather than others trying to speculate what is best for the patient, family members and surgeons can point to a specific document that outlines the individual preferences of the patient. The living will, in this sense, best approximates the standard of promoting the principle of autonomy, as it follows the wishes of the informed, competent patient. When surgeons are treating patients who have life-threatening or terminal illnesses, they initially should appeal to the explicit desires of the patient as laid forth in a living will, if available. Patients have the right to refuse life-sustaining treatment; if he or she clearly has articulated such a desire in a valid living will, these decisions should be honored. Physicians are legally and ethically bound to respect the decisions of patients that are set forth in a living will.

Although living wills are helpful in elucidating a patient's wishes around death and dying, they also suffer from several shortcomings. Living wills require physicians to make decisions on the basis of their interpretation of a written document, rather than an actual discussion with the patient. Situations can, and often do, arise that were not addressed specifically in the living will. In addition, patients who make decisions preemptively often are less informed than patients who are facing a current health problem. Attempts to make living wills less ambiguous by trying to incorporate alternative clinical scenarios are confusing and can be too abstract to be useful to families or surgeons. Because of this, there has been an increasing emphasis on surrogate decision-making.

Every state has a durable-power-of-attorney law that permits patients to designate someone to make decisions for them if they become incapable of doing so for themselves. The *Quinlan* and *Cruzan* cases firmly established the legal and ethical centrality of autonomy and the extension of autonomy through surrogate decision makers. The goal of appointing a proxy is to simplify the process of making decisions by identifying a person—previously chosen by the patient—who can discuss treatment options and has the legal and ethical authority to give or withhold consent on behalf of the patient. In effect, the proxy agent has the authority to make decisions that the patient would have made if he or she were still competent. The agent, however, must make decisions that are consistent with the wishes of the patient, if these are known, and otherwise that are consistent with the patient's best interests.

Only 10% to 20% of patients have completed advanced directives or have identified a proxy decision-maker. Surgeons, therefore, need to be aware of the other mechanisms that are used to identify appropriate courses of action regarding end-of-life issues. These include the best interest standard and substituted judgment. The best interest standard attempts to promote the good of the individual as viewed by the shared values of society. Such factors as the avoidance of death, relief of pain and suffering, preservation or restoration of functioning, and quality and extent of life are usually taken into account [12]. In contrast, substituted judgment occurs when an actual surrogate—not predetermined by the patient as with a health care proxy—attempts to determine what the currently incompetent patient would have decided, had that patient been able to choose. This can be used only if the patient was, at one time, capable of developing preferences and values, and left reliable evidence of those attitudes concerning their current medical condition, such as a discussion of end-of-life decisions with a spouse or other family members [13].

Physicians do not always follow patient or surrogate requests. In one study, 34% of physicians continued life-sustaining treatment, despite patient or surrogate wishes that it be discontinued. In addition, 42% withheld or withdrew life-sustaining treatment unilaterally because they judged additional interventions futile [12,14]. In deliberating on whether to "let a patient go," the principle of autonomy dictates that the wishes of the patient directly, and through their surrogates indirectly, take a prima facie, although not absolute, precedence over the physician's opinion. Although surgeons should not be forced to act against their conscience, they also should realize that withholding or withdrawing life-sustaining therapy is entirely compatible with the ethical principles of autonomy, beneficence, nonmaleficence, and justice.

Ethical distinctions at the end of life

Withholding and withdrawing treatments

Traditionally, there has been much debate around the omission-commission distinction, especially the distinction between withholding and withdrawing treatments. Many clinicians, family members, and patients strongly believe that such a distinction exists ethically and legally. For example, many physicians feel ethically justified in withholding treatments that they never started, but not in withdrawing treatments that already were initiated. Physicians find it easier to limit resuscitative efforts, such as chest compressions, defibrillation, or antiarrhythmic therapy, rather than to withdraw life-sustaining treatments, such as mechanical ventilation, nutrition, or hydration [15]. Physicians also prefer to withdraw forms of therapy that support organs that failed for natural reasons, rather than iatrogenic factors, and to withdraw recently instituted, rather than long-standing, interventions [16]. Medical caregiver discomfort about withdrawing life-sustaining treatment may reflect the view that such actions render them more responsible, and thus, more culpable, for the patient's death. The ethical haziness that surrounds the distinction between withholding and withdrawing treatment can lead to management that is inappropriate and may delay more fitting palliative measures.

Most ethicists have concluded that the distinction between withholding and withdrawing treatment is morally incoherent. Treatment always can be withdrawn permissibly if it can be withheld permissibly [5]. This permits the possibility of taking a potentially life-saving step without being forbidden to reverse the decision if it proves, with further information or time, to have been the wrong choice [1]. This moral acceptability is crucial in making treatment decisions in the face of the prognostic uncertainty that surgeons face every day. Surgeons should be morally free to make clinical treatment decisions on the basis of available knowledge, not discomfort and uncertainty that a current decision is "irreversible." The moral irrelevance of the distinction between withholding and withdrawing treatment allows surgeons to make decisions without being burdened by the potential that they cannot stop a trial intervention when the patient's interests are no longer served by it. If surgeons make decisions using the irrelevant distinction between withholding and withdrawing, the surgeon may even be morally culpable for burdening patients with extended suffering. The distinction between withholding and withdrawing treatment does not provide an ethical justification for prolonging a patient's clinical course that will end inevitably in death.

Ordinary and extraordinary treatments

In the past, some individuals have held the belief that the failure to supply ordinary means of preserving life is equivalent to euthanasia. The distinction between ordinary and extraordinary treatments has been cited widely to justify or to condemn decisions around life-sustaining treatments. Traditionally, extraordinary treatments were seen as being ethically unnecessary, but ordinary treatments could not be foregone legitimately. The distinction between ordinary and extraordinary means has had a long tradition in medical practice, legal decisions, and, in particular, Roman Catholic moral theology [17,18].

The terms "ordinary" and "extraordinary" are difficult to define but the general concept behind each term can be characterized. "Ordinary" usually refers to those means that that can be obtained and used without great difficulty and that offer a reasonable hope of benefit without excessive pain or other inconvenience. In contrast, "extraordinary" usually refers to those means that involve excessive difficulty, cannot be obtained without excessive pain or inconvenience, and which, if used, do not offer necessarily a reasonable hope of benefit [5,18]. These definitions provide little moral guidance. Ordinary or extraordinary only can be determined in reference to the individual, and the categories themselves say nothing about the duties of medical professionals. Virtually all treatment interventions are sometimes burdensome and sometimes helpful. Reasonable surgeons also often can disagree on what constitutes "a reasonable hope of benefit." Therefore, the distinction between ordinary and extraordinary is vague and ethically untenable.

The principal consideration of any treatment should be whether it is beneficial or burdensome, not whether it falls into the artificial category of ordinary or extraordinary. For example, the "ordinary" means of intravenous fluids and nutrition may be unduly burdensome to a patient who is in a persistent vegetative state who previously articulated that he would not want to be sustained in such a condition. In contrast, the "extraordinary" means of high-dose vasopressors and hemodialysis may be morally justifiable in a patient who strongly desires "heroic measures." The moral distinction of ordinary versus extraordinary care, therefore, is conceptually incoherent, and in practice, unhelpful. As such, the termination of gastrointestinal feedings and intravenous fluids may, at times, be morally acceptable. In making such end-of-life decisions, the surgeon should not focus on whether an intervention is ordinary or extraordinary. Instead, surgeons should determine how the intervention in question impacts the patients quality-of-life—what are the benefits and the burdens of the treatment to the specific patient that lies before you?

Futile care

Sometimes, surgeons are faced with patient- or family-driven requests for overtreatment—the providing of certain interventions or surgical procedures that in the surgeon's best clinical estimation would not result in a benefit to the patient. The area of providing "futile" care remains controversial. Some ethicists believe that it always is the patient's (or family's) right to determine what is medically appropriate for each particular patient and that the surgeon never has the right to determine unilaterally that an intervention is inappropriate. Other ethicists believe that futile care is ethically unjustifiable, as it holds autonomy (the patient's right to choose) as an absolute in all situations and ignores other valid principles, such as nonmaleficence (ie, performing a procedure that may cause pain but has no clinical benefit) and justice (ie, providing a service that is of no benefit at the cost of society).

The term "futile" eludes definition. In essence, a futile action is one that cannot achieve the goals that are intended by the action, no matter how often it is repeated. It denotes an action that will fail and that ought not be attempted [19]. If futile treatment is defined as treatment that can no longer be expected to achieve beneficial ends, the question becomes "what is a reasonable level of expectation and who defines what constitutes beneficial ends?". In this sense, futility has two aspects—one quantitative and the other qualitative [19]. Quantitative futility focuses on the probability that a particular outcome can be achieved and involves the judgment that once this probability falls below a threshold, it is not worth pursuing (ie, it is futile). A defined rate of success below which care would be deemed futile has never been agreed on and is fraught with problems of ambiguity and arbitrariness [20]. This brings us to the second aspect of futility, the qualitative dimension. Describing a therapy as futile incorporates a value judgment that carrying out the therapy is not worth it (ie, usefulness or futility only can be judged relative to an end). The question then becomes "who decides whether the quality of life that is associated with a certain medical treatment is futile?". Such a discussion is particularly important because physicians consistently judge patients' quality of life to be significantly lower than how patients judge their own quality of life.

The concept of medical futility, therefore, is pragmatically ineffectual and ethically invalid [21]. Although everyone can agree that futile care should be avoided, the term itself cannot be defined universally. The word "futile" connotes a categorical ring that masks the more subtle ethical and clinical complexities that face the surgeon. Given the confusion around the issue of futile care, what is a surgeon to do when faced with a demand for an intervention that he or she believes to be medically inappropriate? The surgeon should discuss the clinical situation with the patient or proxy decision-maker, identify the various therapeutic options, and delineate the reasons why the requested intervention is medically inappropriate. The surgeon also should recommend a second medical opinion. If the second opinion corroborates that the intervention would be futile but the patient or family still does not agree, then the surgeon should seek assistance from the appropriate institutional resources, such as the ethics committee and hospital administration. Although the surgeon is not ethically obligated to provide treatment that he or she believes is futile and that would violate his or her sense of self-integrity, the surgeon is responsible for continued care of the patient, which may involve helping to transfer the patient to a surgeon who is willing to provide the requested intervention [22].

Terminal sedation and the principle of double effect

Pain management and symptom control often is a difficult issue to address in the dying patient and pain management frequently is inadequate in the dying patient [23,24]. One reason for this is that the surgeon often is confronted with the clinical challenge of trying to keep the dying patient comfortable, while also trying to avoid overmedicating the patient. The classic instance where this concern arises is the patient who is short of breath for whom morphine would be palliative but also may depress respiratory drive. Although the surgeon wants to alleviate the patient's pain, he or she also has a justifiable aversion to doing something that may hasten the patient's death.

Clinical situations in which sedation is the proximate cause of patient death are extremely rare. With incremental increases in analgesia, patients usually acclimate to the drug's analgesic and respiratory depressive effects. Despite this, supposing that the surgeon could provide medication to relieve the patient's suffering and that this medication might result in a substantial risk that the patient would die earlier as a result, what is the surgeon ethically obligated to do? In such a situation, the concept of double effect often is espoused.

The doctrine of double effect recognizes that an action may have a good and a bad effect. The doctrine of double effect distinguishes between intended effects or consequences and foreseen effects or consequences. For example, under the doctrine of double effect, a physician may provide a medication to relieve suffering that may accelerate death if the surgeon's intent is to relieve suffering and not to hasten death. An action is permissible if the bad effect was merely foreseen, but not intended [25]. The classic formulation of the doctrine of double effect has four elements (Table 2) [5]. Specifically, the act itself cannot be intrinsically wrong and the surgeon has to have the proper intent—the relief of pain and suffering—not the intent of killing the patient. The concept of double effect, however, is controversial and critics argue that the principle is sometimes confusing and difficult to apply. For example, it is not always easy to distinguish the intended from the merely foreseen. Regardless of the problems with the doctrine of double effect, it remains useful as a tool for ethical analysis. The doctrine highlights the importance of proportionality and the importance of minimizing needless suffering and avoiding interventions that are more harmful than beneficial given the patient's overall prognosis.

Killing and letting die: euthanasia and physician-assisted suicide

Like other previously discussed ethical categories, the distinction between assisted death and natural death is vague. However, unlike the other

Table 2
Four classic conditions for the doctrine of double effect [5]

Condition	Definition
1. Nature of the act	Act itself must not be intrinsically wrong, or at least morally neutral.
2. Intention	The person must intend only the good effect. Although the bad effect may be foreseen, it must not be intended.
3. Distinction between means and effect	The good effect is produced directly by the action and not by the bad effect; the bad effect must not be a means to the good effect.
4. Proportionality between good and bad effect	The good effect is sufficiently desirable to compensate for allowing for the bad effect.

distinctions that were noted above (withholding versus withdrawing and ordinary versus extraordinary), the distinction between killing, (ie, physician-assisted death or suicide) and letting die needs to be maintained.

Although some ethicists argue that killing and letting die are morally indistinguishable, we believe that a moral distinction needs to be maintained to differentiate the act of letting a patient die versus the act of being a proximate, direct, and intentional cause of a patient's death. This is not to say that surgeons ethically cannot be indirect agents in hastening a patient's death (eg, removing a patient from a ventilator or giving a patient high-dose narcotics to alleviate pain). Surgeons, however, are not justified by ethical or professional standards to assist purposely or intentionally with the intent of quickening a patient's demise, even if it is deemed to be "merciful." In other words, we believe that physician-assisted suicide (PAS) is not morally justifiable.

One of the most well-known cases that catapulted the issue of PAS into the arena of public debate was that of Timothy Quill and his patient, Diane [26]. The case was one of the first instances of an American physician publicly acknowledging and advocating a role for physicians in assisted suicides. Since the publication of the case in *The New England Journal of Medicine*, the medical, ethical, as well as the broader national community have struggled to articulate a cohesive position on the subject. Undoubtedly, the issue of PAS is complex. It challenges all four of the classic ethical principles. PAS draws strongly on different notions of each of these principles in their support or criticism of PAS. PAS also radically questions our intentions and our virtues, as well as our character as individuals and as a society. Faced with the existential reality of suffering, pain, and death we are forced to provide answers: will we relieve pain? even to the point of causing unintentional death? or is it morally permissible to cause death intentionally to avoid and minimize pain? These questions are not answered easily.

Proponents of PAS characterize it as a compassionate act that is consistent with the physician's professional role as patient advocate. They claim that the purpose of medicine is not to prevent death but to alleviate suffering, and that PAS accomplishes this. From a moral and legal standpoint, the advocates of PAS question the distinction between refusing medical treatment (which enjoys legal sanction) and PAS (which is legally prohibited). "Whether a doctor turns off a respirator in accordance with the patient's request or prescribes pills that a patient may take when he is ready to kill himself, the doctor acts with the same intention: to help the patient die" [27]. Proponents of PAS, therefore, argue that the two acts are morally and legally indistinguishable. The advocates of PAS go beyond the claim that PAS is a social good; they insist that PAS is an individual's right— a voluntary choice by a competent adult should be respected in the name of patient autonomy.

By attempting to make the refusal of medical treatment and assisted suicide similar (if not identical), the practical implication is that both would benefit from the same legal and public policy protections. There are, however, compelling factors to distinguish between refusal of life-sustaining treatment and assisted suicide for law and public policy reasons, despite any similarities on a case-by-case basis.

The New York State Task Force on Life and the Law [28] previously articulated the distinction between refusing medical treatment and PAS. In this document, the committee argues that the refusal of medical treatment needs to be distinguished from PAS on several legal and philosophical points. The initial distinction is a legal one. The right to refuse life-sustaining treatment simply is an application of the long-standing prohibition of battery. The courts, in *Cruzan* and other cases, explicitly grounded the right to refuse treatment in the long-standing right to resist unwanted physical invasions, rather than in a broader right to hasten death. In *Cruzan*, "given the common law rule that forced medication was a battery, and the long legal tradition protecting the decision to refuse unwanted medical treatment, the court's assumption was entirely consistent with this nation's history and constitutional traditions" [29]. The court acknowledged that although the decision to commit suicide may be just as personal as the decision to refuse treatment, it never has enjoyed similar legal protection.

The second distinction between refusal of treatment and PAS concerns the issue of intentionality and causality. PAS supporters assert that in refusal of treatment and PAS the physician acts with the same intention—to help the patient die. By removing a respiratory tube or prescribing lethal pills, the physician causes the patient's death. This argument, however, blurs the finer distinctions that are necessary for legal and ethical deliberations. The determination of causation as a factual matter and the determination of causation for purposes of assessing ethical accountability can be, and need to be, differentiated. To understand this, we must distinguish the object of the physician's activity in the removal of life-sustaining therapy and PAS. To accomplish this, we must examine the principle of cooperation.

Whether a physician removes life-sustaining treatment or provides lethal pills, he or she is, to some degree, cooperating with the object of hastening a patient's death. The principle of cooperation, however, would encourage us to distinguish exactly what the object (intention) of the physician's activity is in each case (similar to the principle of double effect). This principle provides a tool to examine more closely the behavior, action, and cooperation of the physician in each case and to ask if it is justifiable. There are many types and degrees of cooperation. The first is the distinction between formal and material cooperation. In formal cooperation, the agent intentionally aims at bringing about a specific end (eg, death) through his actions. In contrast, in cooperating materially, the agent may acknowledge a variety of different intentions in his actions; however, none is aimed directly at the "undesirable" end, here death. Let us, for example, consider a patient who has a hopeless terminal illness who has her mechanical ventilator support removed by a physician and subsequently dies. Although the physician may be the proximate cause of her death, the ultimate cause is that of the underlying disease. Although the physician has cooperated materially in hastening the patient's death, he or she has not cooperated formally. That is, the physician has not caused the patient's death directly. In contrast to this, let us consider the patient who has the same terminal illness but dies after taking the lethal prescription that was provided to her by her physician. In this instance, the physician is the proximate and ultimate cause of the patient's death. The physician formally has intended the death of the patient. Unlike patients who take lethal drugs, patients who refuse life-sustaining treatment will not die unless they are suffering from an underlying disease process that makes life impossible without medical support. As Daniel Callahan [30] notes, "there must be an underlying fatal pathology if allowing to die is even possible." Thus, with determination of causation in PAS and refusal-of-treatment cases, causation cannot be based solely on empiric observation. Rather, the proximate and ultimate causes, as well as considerations of formal and material cooperation, need to be discriminated. Evaluation of one's actions in light of each of these can lead to different underlying assessments of moral responsibility and legal permissibility.

A detrimental effect of PAS would be its undermining of what it means to be a physician, a medical professional, and a caregiver. The hallmark of the medical profession has always been one of nurturing. The physician unceasingly has been a steadfast advocate for life. This commitment to protecting life, to providing care, and to comforting the ill always has occurred in the context of a loving patient–physician relationship. The prospect of PAS threatens this. Instead of being an advocate for the patient, physicians risk becoming advocates of particular paths—one of which could be death. In adopting PAS as a practice, physicians risk being transformed slowly as professionals, but perhaps more importantly, also as individuals. As Aquinas noted, every human action is a moral action [31]. Any action that we perform knowingly is a moral action because it affects ourselves and others as moral agents, shaping us and what we become. In short, we become what we practice. A person who consistently lies becomes a liar. A person who practices dance becomes a dancer. It is here, then, that one of the greatest perils regarding PAS and the physician resides. If physicians, as individuals and as moral agents, consistently and systematically assist in the killing of their patients what will this ultimately mean? Will this not in some fundamental fashion change the identity and character of the physician as a person? For thousands of years, the profession of medicine has been made up of people who have seen themselves as caregivers and healers. To become involved in the systematic killing of patients, even if for the "right" reasons, nonetheless would change this identity of the physician. Such a fundamental shift in the profession and how we see ourselves as moral agents should not be taken lightly.

When analyzing PAS in more depth, we are reminded of the need to address our social shortcomings, rather than a need to legalize PAS. In a society that undervalues the sick and the suffering, PAS seems hazardous. Rather than adopting PAS, surgeons and society should be motivated to re-examine the manner in which we treat suffering, pain, dying, and death. Instead of the quicker, and perhaps, easier solution of PAS, surgeons must take up the more difficult project of how to be creative, productive, and innovative in the face of suffering and death. Surgeons need to focus more on compassionate care and pain relief. More focus needs to be placed on support structures: medical (eg, patient support groups, physician-patient dialog), social (job support, health leave, family support), and financial (innovative payment and insurance plans). In short, we need to learn how to reach out more effectively to those who are in need at the end of life. We need to challenge ourselves as surgeons and as caregivers to create, to build, and to find a place for those in need.

References

[1] Danis M, Federman D, Fins JJ, et al. Incorporating palliative care into critical care education: principles, challenges, and opportunities. Crit Care Med 1999;27(9):2005–13.
[2] Mosenthal AC, Lee KF, Huffman J. Palliative care in the surgical intensive care unit. J Am Coll Surg 2002;194(1):75–83 [discussion 84–5].
[3] Prendergast TJ, Luce JM. Increasing incidence of withholding and withdrawal of life support from the critically ill. Am J Respir Crit Care Med 1997;155(1):15–20.
[4] Smedira NG, Evans BH, Grais LS, et al. Withholding and withdrawal of life support from the critically ill. N Engl J Med 1990;322(5):309–15.
[5] Beauchamp T, Childress J. Principles of biomedical ethics. New York: Oxford University Press; 1994.
[6] Pawlik TM, Platteborze N, Souba WW. Ethics and surgical research: what should guide our behavior? J Surg Res 1999;87(2):263–9.

[7] Hauerwas S. Toward an ethics of character. Theol Stud 1972;33:33–41.

[8] Lynn J, Teno JM, Phillips RS, et al. Perceptions by family members of the dying experience of older and seriously ill patients. SUPPORT Investigators. Study to Understand Prognoses and Preferences for Outcomes and Risks of Treatments. Ann Intern Med 1997;126(2): 97–106.

[9] Faber-Langendoen K. A multi-institutional study of care given to patients dying in hospitals. Ethical and practice implications. Arch Intern Med 1996;156(18):2130–6.

[10] Annas GJ. The health care proxy and the living will. N Engl J Med 1991;324(17):1210–3.

[11] Faber-Langendoen K, Lanken PN. Dying patients in the intensive care unit: forgoing treatment, maintaining care. Ann Intern Med 2000;133(11):886–93.

[12] Nyman DJ, Sprung CL. End-of-life decision making in the intensive care unit. Intensive Care Med 2000;26(10):1414–20.

[13] President's Commission on the Study of Ethical Problems in Medicine and Biomedical and Behavioral Research. Deciding to forego life-sustaining treatment: ethical, medical, and legal issues in treatment decisions. Washington, DC: Government Printing Office; 1983.

[14] Asch DA, Hansen-Flaschen J, Lanken PN. Decisions to limit or continue life-sustaining treatment by critical care physicians in the United States: conflicts between physicians' practices and patients' wishes. Am J Respir Crit Care Med 1995;151(2 Pt 1):288–92.

[15] Dowdy MD, Robertson C, Bander JA. A study of proactive ethics consultation for critically and terminally ill patients with extended lengths of stay. Crit Care Med 1998;26(2):252–9.

[16] Christakis NA, Asch DA. Biases in how physicians choose to withdraw life support. Lancet 1993;342(8872):642–6.

[17] Kelly G. The duty to preserve life. Theol Stud 1951;12:550–6.

[18] Kelly G. The duty of using artificial means of preserving life. Theol Stud 1954;25:203–20.

[19] Schneiderman LJ, Jecker NS, Jonsen AR. Medical futility: its meaning and ethical implications. Ann Intern Med 1990;112(12):949–54.

[20] Youngner SJ. Who defines futility? JAMA 1988;260(14):2094–5.

[21] Hinshaw DB, Pawlik T, Mosenthal AC, et al. When do we stop, and how do we do it? Medical futility and withdrawal of care. J Am Coll Surg 2003;196(4):621–51.

[22] Halevy A, Baldwin JC. Poor surgical risk patients. In: McCullough LB, Jones JW, Brody BA, editors. Surgical ethics. New York: Oxford University Press; 1998. p. 152–70.

[23] Cleeland CS, Gonin R, Hatfield AK, et al. Pain and its treatment in outpatients with metastatic cancer. N Engl J Med 1994;330(9):592–6.

[24] Knaus WA, Harrell FE Jr, Lynn J, et al. The SUPPORT prognostic model. Objective estimates of survival for seriously ill hospitalized adults. Study to understand prognoses and preferences for outcomes and risks of treatments. Ann Intern Med 1995;122(3):191–203.

[25] Arras J, Steinbock B, London AJ. Moral reasoning in the medical context. In: Arras J, Steinbock B, editors. Ethical issues in modern medicine. Mountain View (CA): Mayfield Publishing Co.; 1999. p. 1–40.

[26] Quill TE. Death and dignity. A case of individualized decision-making. N Engl J Med 1991; 324(10):691–4.

[27] Dworkin R, Nagel T, Nozick R, et al. The philosopher's brief. In: Arras J, Steinbock B, editors. Ethical issues in modern medicine. Mountain View (CA): Mayfield Publishing Co.; 1999. p. 258–66.

[28] The New York State Task Force on Life and Law. The distinction between refusing medical treatment and suicide. In: Arras J, Steinbock B, editors. Ethical issues in modern medicine. Mountain View (CA): Mayfield Publishing Co.; 1999. p. 266–73.

[29] Washington v Harold Glucksberg, United States Supreme Court, 1997.

[30] Callahan D. The troubled dream of life: in search of a peaceful death. New York: Simon and Schuster; 1993.

[31] Keenan J. Ten reasons why Thomas Aquinas is important for ethics today. New Blackfriars 1994;75:354–63.

ELSEVIER
SAUNDERS

SURGICAL
CLINICS OF
NORTH AMERICA

Surg Clin N Am 85 (2005) 287–302

Palliative Care: Good Legal Defense

K. Francis Lee, MD, FACS

*Department of Surgery, Baystate Medical Center, Tufts University School of Medicine,
759 Chestnut Street, Springfield, MA 01199, USA*

The perceived risk of legal liability looms large as a major barrier to optimal palliative care among surgeons. Aggressive pain management may cause respiratory depression and death, whereas withdrawal of support may lead to a charge of manslaughter. Long-term chronic pain management with high doses of opioid analgesics may invoke an investigation from the Drug Enforcement Administration (DEA). In the current turmoil of the medical malpractice crisis in which regulations reign, the core tenets of palliative care, such as effective communication and pain relief, may have to yield to the specter of increased legal vulnerability.

Yet the facts point otherwise. Legal considerations reinforce the core principles of palliative care. Review of the literature clearly shows a reassuring trend in the recent decade. Major legal and regulatory entities, such as the U.S. Supreme Court, the state courts, the legislatures, and even the DEA, have espoused and echoed the legal and ethical validity of good palliative care. The best legal defense may be a sound clinical practice that is based on good palliative care. The following is a brief review of some of the salient legal principles and precedents that may be of interest to surgeons who wish to practice good palliative care without the fear of legal liability.

Palliative analgesia and sedation: legal support

When surgeons provide pain relief to patients who have terminal conditions, whether in advanced metastatic malignancy or multi-organ system failure, tension arises at some point between the need to prescribe a higher dose of analgesia and the potential for respiratory depression and hastened death. The fear of the secondary effect of hastened death often

---

The presented material is the author's academic commentary. For expert legal advice, the reader is advised to consult a licensed legal counsel.

E-mail address: francis.lee@bhs.org

restrains the surgeon from prescribing adequate doses of analgesia. This leads to unnecessary pain, even as the patient suffers from a terminal condition.

Based on the principles of double effect and beneficence, the surgeon is not at increased legal risk when the patient's death is the secondary effect of large doses of analgesia to relieve suffering from the terminal condition. The intent to palliate fulfills the ethical goal of beneficence, as long as the intent is clear, evident, and warranted by the clinical situation. The palliative intent must be well-documented, as would be the case with any surgical practice.

The principle of double effect is applicable when an act with the primary intention of doing good produces a secondary effect that is harmful. The doctrine is borne out of a medieval, theologic exegesis of self-defense [1] but has modern legal ramifications. The principle would be operational in terminal sedation when the following four conditions are met: (1) death occurs as a side effect of high-dose analgesia; (2) the attempt at pain relief is indicated clinically and warranted morally; (3) the attempt at pain relief is not achieved mainly by way of death (eg, as in euthanasia or physician-assisted suicide); and (4) the benefit of pain relief is not outweighed by the occurrence of death (which is inevitable in a terminal condition, by definition, and thus alone does not outweigh the harm of unnecessary suffering plus inevitable death) [1].

The U.S. Supreme Court has accepted palliative analgesia and sedation as legally permissible when no other means are available to relieve pain and suffering [2,3]. Chief Justice Rehnquist affirmed the State may "permit palliative care related to (refusal of unwanted lifesaving treatment)...which may have the foreseen but unintended 'double effect' of hastening the patient's death" [2].

The rulings have rejected euthanasia as being an unlawful activity in every U.S. jurisdiction, and further argued that under circumstances in which palliative measures are available, there is no constitutional right to physician-assisted suicide. Significantly, the Court distinguished both acts from palliative sedation, which it deemed as legal and ethical.

Legal action that involves palliative analgesia and terminal sedation and leads to unanticipated death is an exceptionally rare occurrence. Only a handful of cases is available for review; a careful examination of them leaves the legal-minded surgeon more reassured than threatened. In the most pertinent and publicized case of *State v Weitzel* [4], a psychiatrist initially was convicted in 1998 on two counts of manslaughter and three counts of negligent homicide in the deaths of five elderly patients after they received large doses of morphine. In 2001, however, a retrial was granted when it was discovered the prosecutors wrongfully withheld the opinions of their own expert witness, who noted "the principle of double effect was applicable" [4]. The witness also opined the treatments rendered were "good faith attempts at comfort care" that did not warrant criminal prosecution [4]. In 2002, the 2nd Judicial District Court of Utah found the psychiatrist not guilty on all counts.

In *State v Naramore* [5], the physician administered increasing amounts of intravenous fentanyl and Versed to a 78-year-old woman who suffered from unrelenting cancer pain. The family discussed the patient's living will, which called for avoidance of "heroic measures" and requested adequate analgesia. When the son refused opioid dosages that might "speed her death," the physician no longer wanted to be involved in the case. The patient was transferred to another facility where she died a couple of days later, presumably from her cancer. The physician/defendant was charged with attempted murder for fentanyl overdose.

Dr. Naramore also was involved in the care of an 81-year-old man who had an acute stroke with minimal neurologic function who was being sustained by mechanical ventilation. In the terminal course of events, he administered intravenous Norcuron as a "maintenance" paralytic dose for mechanical ventilation; however, the ventilator was withdrawn 9 minutes later. He was charged with intentional and malicious second-degree murder.

Initially, Dr. Naramore was convicted of attempted murder and second-degree murder involving both patients. The case was appealed. The students of palliative care should examine the appellate court decision carefully. As to the 78-year-old patient, the appellate court specifically states, "one of the key issues involved in this case involves what is known as 'palliative care'". In the majority opinion, the Kansas Medical Society's *amicus* brief that explains palliative care and double effect were discussed explicitly, as well as a citation to the American Medical Association's ethical position: "Thus, a health care provider is ethically permitted, and perhaps even required, to implement pain medication and palliative care, with the consent of the patient or the patient's family, notwithstanding the potential for hastening death" [6].

As to the 81-year old patient's death, the Court discussed the defense lawyer's argument of medical futility, quoting the AMA guideline on the appropriate use of cardiopulmonary resuscitation [7] and a legal precedent that relieves the physician of any obligation to treat when treatments are deemed medically "useless" [8]. The Appellate Court noted "the jury was given no instructions (none were requested) on the very difficult issues of palliative care and what are appropriate resuscitation attempts." It further stated "(reversal of verdict) can occur if a jury ignores a fully supported, reasonable explanation for the defendant's actions which negates criminal guilt" [5]. Finally, it weighed the medical expert opinions, of which there were many on both sides, which failed to produce any medical consensus upon which to convict the defendant of criminal liability "beyond reasonable doubt" [5]. Dr. Naramore was acquitted because of insufficient evidence. The summary cogently suggests that because of the lack of knowledge of palliative care and medical futility, "the jury was not free to disbelieve that there was substantial competent medical opinion in support of the proposition that Dr. Naramore's actions were not only noncriminal, but were medically appropriate" [5].

The final ruling of the Appellate Court aside, *State v Naramore* illustrates interesting legal considerations for palliative care. Careful examination of the case reveals Dr. Naramore's legal troubles were not associated with the practice of palliative care, but rather, originated from the opposite (ie, substandard palliative care). For example, the administration of the paralytic agent, Norcuron, 9 minutes before withdrawal of mechanical ventilation—a basis for the intentional and malicious second-degree murder charge—is a flagrant departure from acceptable palliative care.

Furthermore, there seems to have been a breakdown in communication between the physician and the two families during the course of patient care. The son of the 78-year-old patient suspected that the physician was drawn to what was akin to euthanasia; this became a basis for the attempted murder charge. The refusal of the physician to be involved further in patient care and the transfer of the 78-year-old patient to another facility 2 days before her death did not bode well for the communication and shared decision-making which are important instruments of effective palliative care. With the 81-year-old patient's family, there apparently was a failure to communicate the concepts of medical futility and withdrawal of support sufficiently, as would be expected for a fully informed consent.

The Appellate Court relied heavily on the medical community's *amicus* briefs and expert witness opinions on palliative care, double effect, and medical futility, as well as the fragile balance between the moral obligation to relieve suffering and uncertainties of future clinical outcomes. In the end, the defending physician was acquitted, in part, on the grounds that the jury was not informed about the medical information described above; absent a knowledge of palliative care, they were "not free" to weigh the evidence appropriately.

State v Naramore was tried initially in 1996. In the past 10 years, a significant degree of public education has occurred. Popular ideas, such as patient autonomy and end-of-life care decision-making, are no longer foreign to many care providers or patient groups. There has been a legal trend in the past 10 years toward support of compassionate palliative care for terminal conditions, from the 1997 U.S. Supreme Court rulings to the 1998 reversal of *State v Naramore* and the 2002 reversal of *State v Weitzel*. There have been other legal actions against physicians, but they involved situations that were extraordinary or even bizarre that mostly are irrelevant to the present topic [9–11]. Any surgeon may be sued for any reason at any time; this is un-preventable. Future judicial surprises notwithstanding, the legal trend in the past decade should make surgeons feel more secure as they provide adequate pain relief to those who suffer in the final phases of their terminal illnesses.

Chronic pain management: principle of balance

The caveat is that when prescribing opioid analgesia in significantly high dosages or for unusually long periods, surgeons should not take lightly the associated responsibility and risk. The above legal support for terminal palliation and sedation stands in stark contrast to the momentum with which the law enforcement agencies recently have intensified their investigation and enforcement of controlled substance drugs, especially Oxycontin. For their part, the DEA may be reacting to alarming statistics, such as the more than doubling of emergency department visits, between 1994 and 2001, that were related to narcotic analgesic abuse [12]. Local and national media abound with cases of physicians being investigated or prosecuted by the DEA for alleged criminal activities that involve prescriptions.

Fear and misunderstanding of the laws and regulations that govern the use of opioid prescriptions are well-recognized as reasons for the under-treatment of pain by physicians, in general [13]. It would be easy for surgeons to react to such a climate by choosing to underprescribe pain medications and refer the patient, whenever possible, to pain specialists. It is important for surgeons to learn how to prescribe high dosages of opioid analgesics safely—which may be needed for refractory or malignant pain syndromes—without running the risk of a regulatory offense or legal liability. In most cases, surgeons legitimately refer patients who have chronic postoperative pain syndromes or cancer pain to pain specialists. Not uncommonly, however, surgeons find themselves treating a patient who requires increasing amounts of opioid analgesia. The understanding of a safe, opioid prescription practice sometimes is important to maintain a positive surgeon–patient relationship and to monitor the long-term postsurgical outcome, even when pain specialists are involved.

Surgeons should review some of the recent publications that address how to achieve the "principle of balance," a concept that is endorsed by major palliative care organizations and law enforcement agencies, such as the DEA and the National Association of Attorneys General [14,15]. In particular, the *Frequently Asked Questions and Answers*, written by the DEA and Last Acts Partnership, offers information on the way to prescribe necessary opioid analgesia safely without risking a regulatory or legal problem [14]. According to the "principle of balance," the DEA and the National Association of Attorneys General concur with the palliative care advocates, and assert that medical practice and patient care should not be interfered with or com-promised by efforts to prevent opioid analgesic abuse. The actual incidence of DEA investigation of physicians is rare; 0.075% of all physicians who are registered with the DEA were investigated in 2003. Of these investigations, most involved physicians who are no longer licensed to practice medicine (72.7% of sanctions) [12].

As with the topic of terminal sedation that was discussed above, surgeons should have little reason to fear with chronic pain management as long as they follow good clinical practice (see Appendix). Documentation is of utmost importance to establish the clinical indication, response to treatment, and valid goals and limits of treatment, which should be reassessed continuously during the treatment. Surgeons must monitor for the behaviors that are potential indicators of opioid misuse and abuse. Review of the circumstances that trigger the law enforcement investigation suggests that most surgeons who are in responsible practice settings have no cause for concern. Surgeons should not feel restricted in their attempts to prescribe adequate opioid analgesia to patients who legitimately need them. In the end, the goals of the DEA and physicians are one and the same (ie, adequately relieving pain and suffering while minimizing the risk of misuse and abuse).

Surgeon–patient communication: palliative care skill and legal defense

The principles of palliative care coincide with some of the basic legal precepts. Patient autonomy, adequate disclosure, and surgeon–patient communication dictate a good clinical practice and successful legal defense.

Patient autonomy

This is an ethical and legal principle held in almost every major legal case that involves palliative care. Those who have the capacity to decide have the constitutional right to make informed decisions about their own medical care. Who determines the patient's capacity? The physician has the right and the responsibility to determine if the patient has the ability to understand the benefits, risks, and alternative treatments so as to make a decision. The courts have weighed heavily in favor of the patient's capacity to decide. For example, inability to talk (mechanical ventilation), alcohol consumption, opioid analgesia, mental illness, and "irrational behavior," in and of themselves, do not constitute an incapacity. In addition, capacity may vary from day to day; a previously incapable person may recover the capacity to decide as his medical condition improves. Whereas advance directives and living wills are written documents, they may be revoked at any moment by verbal expressions to the contrary; the changes in the patient's decision must be respected by the care providers.

Patient autonomy is served best by effective communication—a key principle in palliative care—between the surgeon and the patient. In-attention or frank dismissal of the patient's wishes when associated with a bad outcome is a recipe for a medical battery charge. This is a tort that is based on the long-established patient's right to bodily integrity: "every human being of adult years and sound mind has a right to determine what shall be done with his own body and a surgeon who performs an operation without his patient's consent commits an assault for which he is liable in damages" [16]. The surgeon may be held liable if the act is intentional and harmful contact was made, even if the "contact" is indirect or includes prescription drugs or mechanical ventilation [17,18].

Advance directive

In cases in which the patient is incompetent, an advance directive (living will) that dictates the patient's wishes must be honored. The patient's wishes, when explicitly stated in the advance directive, cannot be disregarded or countermanded by the physician or the health care proxy. In the case of a patient with a complicated family situation who is about to undergo a high-risk surgery, the surgeon strongly may consider recommending a preoperative advance directive. Far from frightening the patient, a preoperative discussion of the patient's end-of-life preferences of treatment facilitates a genuine understanding on the part of the surgeon and the future surrogates. Furthermore, a documented advance directive serves as a clear guide to a potentially complex and difficult postoperative decision-making process if an undesirable, life-threatening complication occurs. This eases the stress for the surgeon and the family surrogate if a consensus is not reached.

Health care power-of-attorney

In the case of an incompetent patient, a health care power-of-attorney (HCPA) serves as a decision-making surrogate, often designated as part of the advance directive form. In most states, the HCPA grants its designee the full authority on behalf of the patient to consent to or refuse care. As became evident in the cases of *Cruzan* and *Wendland*, in some states the HCPA does not have the authority to direct a discontinuation of artificial feeding and hydration (leading to patient's death) without an advance directive or other "clear and convincing" evidence of such wishes on the part of the patient [19,20]. The courts strive to ensure the holder of the HCPA acts according to the patient's wishes, if known, and otherwise "in the best interests of the patient." In the case of contradiction, the patient's advance directive overrides the wishes of the surrogate decision-maker. A previously incompetent patient whose clinical recovery returns her capacity can revoke her earlier advance directive or HCPA, either verbally or in writing [21]. For surgeons who frequently engage in high-risk procedures for critical surgical diseases, it would serve them well, if appropriate, to encourage the patient to establish an HCPA and an advance directive. This effective communication of end-of-life care preferences is an important aspect of good palliative care.

When there is no advance directive and no one designated by an HCPA, as in the cases of many patients who require surgical care (often in emergency situations), the surrogate decision-making falls to family members, or in some states, close friends [21]. Generally, the common order is spouse, followed by adult children, parents, siblings, and finally, siblings' adult children [21]. Surgeons should be familiar with their own state's rules regarding surrogate determination, especially when there is a conflict between a long-lost, distant relative and a close friend or partner. In case of emergency, when there is no surrogate available, the surgeon must make reasonable inquiries, but does not have to go to outlandish lengths. Such "reasonable" efforts at reaching a surrogate decision-maker should be documented in the chart along with other clinical information, such as the indication and nature of the emergent surgical intervention and the incapacity of the patient.

Surgeon–patient communication

An advance directive, HCPA, and surrogate decision-making are legal vehicles to respect and ensure patient autonomy in medical care. Even when they are present and used, the patient's autonomy to choose is compromised unless there is adequate disclosure of information. What constitutes adequate informed consent follows one of three approaches: What would a reasonable physician disclose in a similar situation? What would an average patient need to know to make an informed decision in a similar situation? What would the specific patient need to know in the specific case to make an informed decision? Most states have specific judicial precedents or legislative acts that determine the required standard for fully disclosed informed consent. It may be of interest for surgeons to become familiar with the legal requirements of their own state, because the courts continue to confuse the medical community by rendering different standards on a state-by-state basis regarding what constitutes adequate disclosure during informed consent; considerable controversy remains.

In general, effective communication and shared decision-making—core principles in palliative care—are key to minimizing legal exposure. Understanding the patient's or surrogate's need for pertinent clinical information so as to choose among alternatives, addressing their wishes for effective pain relief and other symptom management, and complying with their end-of-life decisions are important facets to effective communication.

Quality of life and pain relief have become increasingly important in today's medical care. First, due to the Joint Commission of Accredited Hospital Organizations' mandate, pain scores are now recorded in medical charts as a "fifth" vital sign [22]. Second, outcomes-based clinical guidelines and professional organizational standards for adequate pain relief are easily accessible to the surgical practitioners, either through the traditional print media or the Internet. Third, the increase of pain specialists and pain treatment centers have increased the availability and expectation of adequate pain management. These three "converging forces" [23] are setting new standards for pain management for the surgeons who often cause or treat perioperative pain. The public's expectation, by and large, eventually finds its voice through jury verdicts. Furrow [23] stated, "tort liability can now build on this convergence in pain management standards."

Failure to communicate with the patient and flagrantly mistreating perioperative pain increasingly may open doors for legal action against the surgeon. Sporadic legal precedents of substandard care of pain have been described previously [21]. Physicians have been found guilty of medical malpractice [24], negligent infliction of emotional distress [25], abandonment [26,27], and elder abuse [28]. A range of legal doctrines that is applicable to substandard pain management has been detailed in the legal literature [29,30].

Surgeons who lack the constitution or the expertise to deal with chronic refractory pain should consider referring the patient to pain specialists. For example, in *Johnson v Kokemoor*, the Supreme Court of Wisconsin recently ruled that the involved surgeon's lack of experience and expertise is "material" information that is admissible in court [31]. The Court held that the surgeon's inexperience should have been disclosed adequately to the patient as part of informed consent, and affirmed that the surgeon should have offered the alternative of referring the patient to a more experienced surgeon at a tertiary medical center. This line of reasoning should be read in conjunction with the opinion in *Freeman v Cleveland Clinic Foundation*; even when the court did not find the defending physician liable for the "proximate cause" of the patient's death, it did not reject the physician's duty to refer the patient to a pain management clinic [32]. These legal considerations suggest that it is in the best interest of the surgeons to examine carefully their sensitivity to patient pain complaints; learn to evaluate, treat, and communicate on various surgical pain syndromes; and align with a capable pain management team to which the refractory cases may be referred easily. In addition, the possibility of chronic debilitating pain should be part of the risks that are communicated to the patient during the preoperative discussion of procedures (eg, inguinal herniorraphy, thoracotomy).

Furthermore, nonsurgical treatment options for seemingly surgical conditions may be an important disclosure during informed consent. Surgeons often do not offer a nonsurgical palliation of pain and symptoms as an alternative to the surgical option. "Surgery or death" has been the customary paradigm of the informed consent for many emergent surgical procedures; however, this "judicial deference to customary practice may be weakening" in face of new clinical management standards [23]. There are circumstances in which quality of life and personal dignity are more important than living-at-all-cost to the patients and surrogates. This may be the case when there are one or more combinations of advanced age, Alzheimer's disease, advanced malignancy, severe congenital neurologic deficit, severely symptomatic end-stage organ system failure, and so forth. In such cases, a nonsurgical palliation of pain and other symptoms may be more aligned with the patient's and surrogate's treatment preferences. Therefore, withholding a discussion of alternative palliative therapy during the preoperative period may constitute inadequate informed consent for which the surgeon may be held liable. In *Branom v State*, failure to discuss the possibility of palliative care as an alternative to surgery was the basis for the legal action against a neonatologist. The plaintiffs were the parents of a newborn who had microcephaly who were "led" to consent to surgery without the discussion of other palliative alternatives [33]. As long as palliative care for certain clinical situations generally is accepted within the surgical community as feasible, legal precedents indicate that surgeons should include palliative modalities—surgical or nonsurgical—as part of a disclosed informed consent [34,35].

Similarly, withdrawal of support should be considered a form of "procedure," and as such, deserves a full informed consent discussion with the surrogate decision-maker. Information to be discussed includes reasonable alternatives to the decision to withdraw support; a detailed description of the steps to discontinue the mechanical ventilation; potential side-effects or complications (including the uncertainties of what may happen following removal of an endotracheal tube); steps that will be taken to minimize adverse events, such as respiratory distress or involuntary muscular movements; and questions asked to confirm adequate understanding by the surrogate decision-maker. These communication steps are good palliative care practice and may minimize the potential occurrence of misunderstanding and legal action. A careful review of *State v Naramore* clearly demonstrates that poor communication during withdrawal of support and terminal sedation largely were responsible for the charges [5].

The days are gone when opioid analgesics are withheld from a dying patient out of legal fears, or paternalistic surgical decisions are made with or without the family consent. The current medical malpractice crisis will not tolerate—judicially or economically—the care providers' overt failures to communicate with patients or to relieve their pain. The above considerations indicate that the legal precepts support—rather than threaten—the principles of palliative care. A recent law that was passed in California recognized "benevolent gestures reduce lawsuits and encourage settlements by fostering the use of apologies in connection with accident-related injuries or death" [36]. Attitudes and actions that demonstrate empathy, compassion, and condolence—"benevolent gestures"—are fundamental palliative skills of a surgeon who cares for the bereavement needs of the family. The new section in the California Evidence Code makes all benevolent gestures by the physician inadmissible evidence in the medical malpractice court. The legislator who authored the new law believed that a simple apology—without admission of guilt—has a positive effect on the overall resolution of a legal dispute [37]. Even the legal system is beginning to understand that good palliative care is good defense against the current medico-legal challenges.

Appendix

The following has been excerpted from Prescription Pain Medications: Frequently Asked Questions and Answers for Health Care Professionals and Law Enforcement Personnel, written collaboratively among the Drug Enforcement Administration, Last Acts Partnership, and Pain & Policy Studies Group of University of Wisconsin [12].

What should be documented when prescribing opioids?

Requirements for documentation when prescribing opioids for the treatment of pain vary from state to state, but several features are endorsed commonly:

The medical record should have evidence that the treatment is taking place within the standards of medical practice.

> For an initial evaluation, this includes a history and physical examination, a pain assessment, and a treatment plan.
> For follow-up visits, this includes an appropriate interim history and focused examination when indicated, pain reassessment, and re-evaluation of the treatment plan.

The medical record should reveal evidence that the physician has evaluated the nature of the pain complaint, earlier treatments, impact of the pain, important comorbidities, and alcohol and drug history.

The medical record should show that a range of outcomes have been repeatedly assessed during the course of opioid therapy, including:

> Pain intensity
> Physical and psychosocial functioning
> Side effects of therapy
> Drug use behaviors (ie, whether any problematic behaviors occur)

The Federation of State Medical Boards of the United States' "Model Policy for the Use of Controlled Substances for the Treatment of Pain" provides more detailed direction on documentation (http://www.fsmb.org). State requirements can be obtained from your state medical board (directory provided at http://www.fsmb.org); state pain policies for each state and can be found at http://www.medsch.wisc.edu/painpolicy/matrix.htm.

How can clinicians assess for risks of abuse, addiction, and diversion and manage their patients accordingly?

Some patients engage in aberrant drug-related behavior during treatment with an opioid or another controlled substance prescription drug. In some cases, this abuse is minor and transitory, whereas in others, it is serious and persistent. Clinicians should recognize that these behaviors may have several causes, including addiction. It is recommended that clinicians adopt a "universal precautions" approach to the use of potentially abusable drugs, including opioids, as discussed below. This approach monitors behaviors over time and structures prescribing that is consistent with the degree of risk of abuse, addiction, and diversion. By establishing treatment expectations for each patient and structuring therapy appropriately, physicians can identify patients who are at risk for abuse, addiction, or diversion; help those who may need controls to manage the therapy responsibly; and provide the monitoring that is needed for safe and effective prescribing.

Clinicians should consider the following approaches in developing a "universal precautions" approach:

In assessing patients for opioid therapy, take a detailed history and perform an appropriate physical examination. The medical history should include a history of controlled prescribed drug use and alcohol, cannabis, and nicotine use. Screen for addictive behaviors of other family members. Take into consideration any social, psychologic, or work-related factors that may indicate a potential for abuse, addiction, or diversion. Identify concurrent psychiatric illness, especially where poor impulse control is a feature.

Establish diagnoses for the pain problem and for relevant comorbidities, and record these in the chart. Base the diagnosis on appropriate evaluations and review of patient records, if available. A patient's unwillingness to allow contact with previous providers should be evaluated and documented.

Consider multiple approaches to the treatment of chronic pain. Nonpharmacologic and nonopioid analgesic approaches may be preferred. Some states have special requirements for treatments that should be tried before opioids.

Consider opioid therapy for all patients who have chronic moderate to severe pain, but evaluate the answers to the following questions first and make case-by-case decisions about the appropriateness of an opioid trial:

What is conventional medical practice in the treatment of this type of pain?

Are there other treatments that are effective and feasible and have a risk-to-benefit profile as good as or better than opioids?

Is the patient particularly vulnerable to opioid side effects?

Is the patient likely to take medications responsibly or, if problems seem likely, could a plan for structuring the therapy and monitoring it be successful?

Recognize that opioid therapy is as much a "therapeutic trial" as any other treatment. If the benefits are not clear or if the risks of adverse effects are not managed easily, the therapy can be modified or stopped.

One practitioner should have primary responsibility for management of chronic pain in patients who have a known or suspected history of abuse, addiction, or diversion.

When a patient has a known history of abuse, addiction, or diversion, it is particularly important that the clinician be clear from the beginning about expectations in the treatment plan. The treatment plan may include a written agreement with the patient that describes the requirements (eg, limited quantities of medication, routine urine screens, consultation with a specialist) and the consequences of not adhering to the agreement.

If the clinician decides to initiate opioid therapy, it is appropriate to begin by titrating the amount of opioid to ensure that maximum therapeutic effect can be reached. Continuation of therapy is justified if the benefit is demonstrably greater than the adverse outcomes; this should be documented clearly. After adequate pain relief has been achieved, a successfully treated patient is one who remains responsible over time, follows the agreement for use of the opioids and exhibits neither drug abuse behaviors nor indications of addiction, and experiences enhanced comfort and improved quality of life. At the other extreme, patients who manifest the disease of addiction exhibit a range of maladaptive behaviors and experience a decreased quality of life. They do not follow the agreement for use of opioids; do not conform to the agreed-upon dosing schedule; and may lose prescriptions, repeatedly seek early refills, or obtain additional supply from other sources. They continue or escalate medication use despite adverse consequences; seem to be unaware of, or in denial about, abuse of the medication; and may have a "story." In some cases, such a patient will "doctor shop" or alter prescriptions to increase his or her supply of the medication.

A "universal precautions" approach to the prescribing of controlled prescription drugs does not mean that all patients who have the capacity to engage in abuse or diversions will be identified, or prevented from these behaviors over time. Nonetheless, the approach emphasizes the value of ongoing assessment and close monitoring, which are essential aspects to the appropriate, safe, and effective use of these over time.

Under what circumstances will the federal Drug Enforcement Administration investigate and prosecute a doctor or pharmacist of refer cases to other agencies?

According to the DEA, most DEA-registered practitioners are honest, ethical people who strive to satisfy their legal and regulatory responsibilities. The target of the DEA complaint investigations is the small number of practitioners who operate with criminal intent. For a physician to be convicted of illegal sale, the authorities must show that the physician knowingly and intentionally prescribed or dispensed controlled substances outside of the scope of the legitimate practice.

The DEA focuses its limited manpower and resources on the flagrant violators. To understand the DEA's intent and practices, it is important to keep in mind that:

State and local agencies, including licensing boards, police departments, Medicaid fraud units, etc., also conduct investigators related to controlled substance diversion, fraud, or improper medical practice.

The DEA investigates a small number of physicians (eg, during fiscal year 2003, the DEA initiated a total of 732 investigations concerning doctors, 584 of which resulted in some form of sanction. In short, approximately 0.075% of all physicians who are registered with the DEA were the subject of some type of DEA investigation during the year).

A significant number of these investigations were initiated because the physician in question was no longer licensed to practice medicine, and therefore, was no longer entitled to DEA registration. In 424 such cases, the physicians elected to surrender the DEA registrations. This represents 72.7% of the 584 "sanctions" that were imposed by the DEA. In 34 cases, the physician's DEA registration was revoked.

During fiscal year 2003, the DEA arrested 50 physicians whose activities were deemed to be knowingly and intentionally beyond the scope of medical practice (ie, criminal). This represents 0.005% of physician registrants.

Most frequently, the DEA responds to complaints, allegations of diversion, or some other impropriety. Depending on the content, most of these are referred to state medical boards or local police.

Joint investigations may occur when local police and state or federal agencies seek out the DEA for its expertise.

The DEA does use administrative sanctions (eg, letters of admonition, memoranda of understanding) rather than criminal investigations when the complaint or allegation relates to such activities as faulty record keeping. Of the 584 actions mentioned above that were taken during fiscal year 2003, 67 were of this nature.

Following receipt of information concerning a physician or pharmacist, an investigator makes inquiries to ascertain the validity of the allegation. Practitioners should be aware that a preliminary inquiry does not mean necessarily that wrongdoing has occurred. The nature of the inquiry varies based on the type of information received. For example, if the allegation pertains to a doctor who prescribes controlled substances without conducting medical examinations, the investigator would be required to obtain information about the doctor's prescribing habits. In the absence of a prescription-monitoring program, investigators would be required to visit pharmacies to review prescription files. If the complaint pertained to a pharmacist, a review of the pharmacy's prescriptions, and possibly, an audit, would be conducted.

An investigation that uncovers inappropriate activity may be resolved through a variety of administrative, civil, or criminal actions. Factors that are considered when law enforcement personnel are determining what action to take include the opinion of medical experts, the egregiousness of the violations, and whether the practitioner is believed to have engaged in the violation knowingly or intentionally. The legal system does not allow practitioners to disregard consciously indications that illegal drug-related activities might be occurring.

A DEA criminal investigation may involve a search warrant, but only if the DEA has sufficient evidence to convince a federal judge or magistrate that it is warranted. Although a search is not a charge and may not result in an arrest, it is a serious matter; normal police protocol involves control of the premises and safety of the participants.

Generally, cases would be referred to other agencies if a practitioner's activities are found to be outside of the course of professional practice, but not significant enough to warrant federal prosecution.

Do the number of patients in a practice who receive opioids, the number of tablets prescribed for each patient, or the duration of therapy with these drugs indicate abuse or diversion?

The number of patients in a practice who receive opioids, the number of tablets that is prescribed for each patient, and the duration of therapy with these drugs do not, by themselves, indicate a problem, and they should not be used as the sole basis for an investigation by regulators or law enforcement. These factors, combined with others, may indicate that prescriptions are being issued or dispensed for other than legitimate medical purposes or not in the course of professional practice.

Characteristics of practitioner or pharmacy that warrant further inquiry that could lead to an investigation include:

A large proportion of prescriptions being paid for in cash.

Large distances between the doctor, patients, and pharmacy, particularly if a sizable proportion of a doctor's prescriptions are being filled at a pharmacy that is not located conveniently to the doctor or the patients.

Drugs and dosages being prescribed are not individualized.

One physician writing multiple prescriptions for numerous patients that are filled consecutively in one pharmacy, indicating that either one person is presenting multiple prescriptions, or several people are filling similar prescriptions at the same time.

A high frequency of prescriptions to replace lost prescriptions or medications.

Frequent premature renewal or refilling of prescriptions.

Frequent prescribing of unusual combinations of drugs, such as stimulants and depressants.

References

[1] Connell FJ. "Double Effect, Principle of". New Catholic Encyclopedia, vol. 4. New York: McGraw-Hill; 1967.
[2] Vacco v Quill, 521 US 793 (1997).
[3] Washington v Glucksberg, 521 US 702 (1997).
[4] State v. Weitzel, Case No. 991700983. Memorandum Decision and Order, Judge Thomas L. Kay, The Second Judicial District Court of Utah, July 1, 2001.
[5] State v Naramore, 965 P.2d 211 (Kan. Ct. App. 1998).
[6] American Medical Association Council on Ethical and Judicial Affairs. Euthanasia: report C. Proceedings of the House of Delegates of the AMA. Chicago: 1988. p. 258–60.

[7] American Medical Association Council on Ethical and Judicial Affairs. Guidelines for the appropriate use of do-not-resuscitate orders. JAMA 1991;265:1868.

[8] Barber v Superior Court of Los Angeles County, 147 Cal. App. 3d 1006, 1018, 195 Cal. Rptr. 484 (1983).

[9] United States v Wood, 207 F.3d 1222 (10th Cir 2000).

[10] People v Schade, 32 Cal. Rptr. 2d 59 (Cal. Ct. App. 1994).

[11] Gilbert v State, 487 So. 2d 1185 (Fla. Dist. Ct. App. 1986).

[12] Drug Enforcement Administration. LastActs, Pain & Policy Studies Group University of Wisconsin. Prescription pain medications: frequently asked questions and answers for health care professionals and law enforcement personnel. Available at: http://www.stoppain.org/faq.pdf. Accessed August 31, 2004.

[13] Fujimoto D. Regulatory issues in pain management. Clin Geriatr Med 2001;17(3):537–51.

[14] Drug Enforcement Administration and 21 Health Organizations Promoting pain relief and preventing abuse of pain medications: a critical balancing act. Available at: http://www.medsch.wisc.edu/painpolicy/dea01.htm. Accessed August 31, 2004.

[15] National Association of Attorneys General. Improving end-of-life care: the role of Attorneys General. Washington, DC: National Association of Attorneys General; 2003.

[16] Schloendorff v Society of New York Hospital, 105 N.E. 92 (N.Y. 1914).

[17] Mink v University of Chicago, 460 F. Supp. 713 (N.D. Ill. 1978).

[18] Leach v Shapiro, 469 NE2d 1047 (Ohio App., 1984).

[19] Cruzan v Director, Missouri Department of Health, 497 US 261 (1990).

[20] Conservatorship of Wendland. 110 Cal. Rptr. 2001;2d:412.

[21] Baluss ME, Lee KF. Legal considerations for palliative care in surgical practice. J Am Coll Surg 2003;197(2):323–30.

[22] Pain assessment and management standards—hospitals. JCAHO Requirement. Standard RI.1.2.9: Patients have the right to appropriate assessment and management of pain. Standard PE.1.4: Pain is assessed in all patients. Available at: http://www.jcrinc.com/subscribers/perspectives.asp?durki=3243. Accessed on August 31, 2004.

[23] Furrow BR. Pain management and provider liability: no more excuses. J Law Med Ethics 2001;29:28–51.

[24] Berger v Sonneland, 26 P3d 257 (WA 2001).

[25] Lynch v Bryant, (Nos. 91–5667, 91–5683, and 91–6054, 6th Cir, 1993).

[26] Kenney v Piedmont Hospital, 222 SE2d 162 (Ga.App., 1975).

[27] In re Bilder. Oregon State Board of Medical Examiners. Sept. 1, 1999.

[28] Bergman v Eden Medical Center, No. H-205732, 2000 WL 519345 (Cal. Sup. Ct. Alameda City).

[29] Rich BA. The emerging standard of care for pain management. William Mitchell Law Rev 2000;26:1.

[30] Shapiro RS. Health care providers' liability exposure for inappropriate pain management. J Law Med Ethics 1996;24:360.

[31] Johnson v Kokemoor, 545 NW2d 495 (Wis. 1996).

[32] Freeman v Cleveland Foundation, 713 NE2d 33 (1998).

[33] Branom v State, 974 P2d 335 (Wash. Ct. App. 1999).

[34] Teilhaber v Greene, 727 A2d 518 (N.J. Super. Ct. 1999).

[35] Moore v Baker, 989 F2d 1129 (11th Cir. 1993).

[36] California Evidence Code AB. 2804, 2000.

[37] Drake W. "I'm sorry": can a doctor show compassion and sympathy without admitting fault? California Association of Physicians website, CAPsules. Available at: http://www.cap-mpt.com/riskmanagement/sorry.html. Accessed on August 31, 2004.

ELSEVIER
SAUNDERS

Surg Clin N Am 85 (2005) 303–313

SURGICAL
CLINICS OF
NORTH AMERICA

Palliative Care in the Surgical ICU

Anne Charlotte Mosenthal, MD, FACS

Division Surgical Critical Care, New Jersey Medical School,
University of Medicine & Dentistry of New Jersey-University Hospital,
150 Bergen Street, Mezzanine 233, Newark, NJ 07103, USA

Mr. Jones is in the surgical ICU (SICU) on a respirator. This is his third admission to the SICU for ventilator support. Three weeks ago he had a pancreatoduodenectomy for pancreatic cancer and his initial recovery was uneventful; however, on postoperative Day 5 he developed pneumonia, rapid atrial fibrillation, and pancreatic ascites. Despite antibiotics, this progressed to respiratory failure and he was placed on the ventilator. He improved and 1 week later was extubated and transferred to the hospital floor, only to relapse within 24 hours with respiratory failure, sepsis, and renal failure. He was readmitted to the SICU for ventilator support, continuous renal replacement therapy, and antibiotics. He improves over 3 weeks time and is now dialysis-free with adequate renal function; however, ventilator weaning is slow with multiple exacerbations of hypoxia and fever. His family states that because of his advanced age and multiple underlying health problems, the patient would not want to be maintained on "these machines" for the remainder of his life. The patient had communicated these wishes to his physicians before surgery. The nurses suggest that ongoing life support is prolonging the patient's suffering; however, the surgeon notes that the prognosis for cancer survival is excellent, and hopes that with time, better nutrition, and slow ventilator weaning, the patient's multiple organ failure will improve and he will survive to be discharged.

This patient's lingering course exemplifies the dilemmas that are encountered increasingly in the SICU when prognosis is unclear and multiple organ failure waxes and wanes. Is Mr. Jones likely to survive to discharge with an acceptable quality of life? Or will he die in the ICU while receiving mechanical ventilation? If he is likely to die, when should care transition to a palliative approach, if at all? As critical care becomes increasingly sophisticated, these sorts of decisions have become part of standard practice for physicians in the ICU.

E-mail address: mosentac@umdnj.edu

0039-6109/05/$ - see front matter © 2005 Elsevier Inc. All rights reserved.
doi:10.1016/j.suc.2005.01.001   *surgical.theclinics.com*

The ICU traditionally has focused on prolonging survival and curing disease with advanced technology; 10% to 20% of patients in the ICU will die before discharge from the hospital [1]. Among ICU survivors, mortality remains high at 6 months, particularly among the elderly [2]. Moreover, one of five American deaths occurs in the hospital during or after an ICU stay [3]. The landmark Study to Understand Prognoses and Preferences for Outcomes and Risks of Treatment (SUPPORT) study demonstrated that a large proportion of dying patients in ICUs received unwanted life support and therapies with inadequate attention to pain and suffering in the last 3 days of life [4,5]. This occurs despite the fact that in the last decade, medical practice found that most deaths in the ICU are associated with withholding or withdrawal of life support [6,7] These trends suggest that expertise in palliative care is an essential part of the armamentarium of the critical care physician, to ensure pain and symptom management in the ICU and to apply the appropriate principles of withholding or withdrawing of life support.

Although it is increasingly clear that the principles of palliative care must be integrated into the ICU to ensure high-quality end-of-life care, how best to do this is not. The particular nature of critically ill surgical patients, critical care surgeons, and the culture of the ICU brings forth special difficulties in integrating palliative care into critical care. First, although 10% to 20% of patients who are admitted to ICU will die during their hospitalization, it is difficult to know with certainty which ones will do so and when. Just as it is unclear whether Mr. Jones in the aforementioned case study is dying or merely following the natural history of multiple organ failure, it is difficult to predict the actual likelihood of mortality for a specific patient. Many predictive models that have been developed for the ICU (eg, Acute Physiology and Chronic Health Evaluation, Multiple Organ Dysfunction Syndrome, Trauma Injury and Severity Score), although useful for stratifying populations, have not proven to be helpful for clinicians who are faced with making decisions about individual patients. The literature suggests that clinicians rarely use prognostic or predictive scores or models for clinical decision making; even when they are informed of the likelihood of death for a particular patient in the ICU based on such models, they do not make a transition to a palliative approach [5,8]. The culture of the ICU traditionally views mortality and survival as dichotomous variables [9]; often death must be imminent before clinicians will change from a curative treatment plan to a palliative one. For example, physicians decide to withdraw mechanical ventilation when they judge patients to have poor long-term cognitive function or less than a 10% likelihood of survival [10]. The wide range of practices regarding end-of-life care and withdrawal and withholding support in ICUs illustrate how prognostic uncertainty and varied definitions of medical futility affect palliative care in the ICU setting.

Most patients who are admitted to the ICU do not have clear advance directives and are unable to participate in medical decisions; this compounds prognostic uncertainty. Only 5% of patients in the ICU can report their end-of-life preferences, their symptoms, or participate in treatment decisions [6]. Much of the decision-making relies upon family members as surrogates. Often, they do not know their loved ones' preferences, are bereaved themselves, and are ill-prepared to participate in serious end-of-life decisions. Furthermore, neither the family nor the patient knows the attending surgeon or intensivist well.

Lastly, almost all patients who enter the SICU, and the physicians who care for them, arrive with goals for curative intent and assumptions that all that technology has to offer will bring about a positive outcome. When coupled with the prognostic uncertainty that was described above, it becomes difficult to know prospectively for each patient when or if goals of care should become palliative. This challenge to palliative care in the ICU setting can be met in several ways. First, quality care in the ICU must include palliative principles, such as pain and symptom relief and good communication for all patients, not only those who are imminently dying or at the end of life. Data suggest that attention to these areas early in ICU care improves the overall quality of critical care, in general, and facilitates specific decision-making around end-of-life care [11,12]. Second, a large part of palliative care in the ICU requires particular expertise in the transition in goals of care and the ability to accomplish curative and palliative goals, in parallel for the same patient. This transition, in the setting of acute life-threatening illness, defines the inherent difficulties and differences in palliative care in the critical care setting. It often must be done acutely, in a compressed time frame, with incomplete information. To accomplish this transition, physicians must have skill in communication for shared decision-making and identifying goals of care, knowledge of the principles of withdrawal and withholding of life support, and familiarity with grief and bereavement support.

The following sections review the four essential areas of palliative care: communication, withholding and withdrawal of organ systems support, pain and nonpain symptom management, and bereavement support as they apply to the SICU setting.

Communication

Effective communication is the mainstay of quality palliative care in the SICU. The integration of palliative care into the intensive care setting relies on early, effective communication between physicians, nurses, the patient, and family; if done well, this will facilitate later difficult transitions in goals of care and end–of-life decision-making. Several studies showed that families of patients in the ICU value communication, particularly with physicians, as highly as medical care and will rate overall quality of critical care based on communication [12,13]. Communication between health care providers also is important for maintenance of the interdisciplinary team that is required for good palliative care.

Although communication long has been regarded as a nice, but nonessential, part of the practice of medicine, particularly surgery, the recognition of competencies that are expected of professionalism validated communication as an essential skill of the surgeon. More importantly, there is increasing evidence in the literature that communication interventions in the ICU have a significant impact on quality of care, length of stay, and patient and family satisfaction. Lilly et al [11,14] found that a family meeting within 72 hours of admission to the ICU decreased the length of stay. This was particularly effective if discussion specifically addressed the patient's goals of care and time-limited therapies, based on the clinical response of the patient. A randomized, prospective trial that used a different model of ethics consultation on nonbeneficial life support found this to be a useful way to resolve conflicts and avoid the prolonged use of futile life support. Length of stay in the ICU and prolonged mechanical ventilation were decreased after the implementation of ethics consultation [15].

Why these interventions work is not entirely clear, although improved resolution of conflicts is a likely benefit. Conflict around end-of-life care is frequent and arises from different understandings of the prognosis, lack of understanding of the patient's preferences, family grief, and poor communication between all parties. Readiness to accept death as a likely outcome for a patient or willingness to entertain withdrawal of life support follows a different time course for each individual, whether he receives or provides treatment. Nurses may precede physicians in this process [13]. Qualitative data from the SUPPORT study suggest that families must accept death of the patient before they can be ready to accept palliative goals of care [16]. Early communication around admission to the ICU, including support for families, may facilitate end–of-life care and decision-making around withdrawal and withholding of life support [17,18].

Despite the demonstrated importance of communication for palliative care in the ICU setting, there is little evidence about the qualitative aspects of communication and how they affect end-of-life care in the ICU. There is a large body of literature on physician–patient communication, but its applicability to the critical care setting is unclear. The compressed time-frame of surgical critical illness, uncertain prognosis, incapacity of the patient, and reliance on bereaved surrogates significantly alter the nature of the communication. Even with this realization, little is known about which interventions might improve quality of communication. Studies that examined the audiotapes of family conferences in the ICU found a correlation between the amount of time that physicians spend listening and the family's satisfaction with the communication [19]. In the surgical setting, even less has been studied about surgeon's communications skills and attitudes around end of life. One study suggests that the critical care nurse plays an important role as mediator and communicator between surgeon and family in the SICU [20]. Lessons also can be drawn from the SUPPORT study; nurse-facilitated communication intervention with physicians and patients did not change end-of-life care significantly with respect to do not resuscitate orders or withdrawal of life support. Nurse specialists providing routinely updated information to physicians on prognosis and patient preferences was not enough to change practice [5]. Whether this reflected deficiencies in the quality of communication or some other aspect of care remains open to speculation. Despite these inconsistent data, recommendations exist for appropriate communication while providing end-of-life care in the critical care setting. Curtis [12] suggests the following six steps for a family meeting, for a patient who is in the ICU patient, based on a modification from earlier principles adapted to the critical care setting. These include: (1) adequate preparation for the discussion, including proper setting, selection of appropriate members of the team, and timing; (2) assessment of family understanding of the situation; (3) discussion of prognosis; (4) clarification of possible outcomes and goals of care; (5) listen and provide empathetic support; and (6) provide a follow-up plan and recommendations for treatment. Further study is needed to identify specific elements of communication in the ICU, particularly in the surgical setting that may improve outcome.

Withdrawal and withholding of life support

The option of withdrawal and withholding of life support, based on informed patient consent, in the ICU is considered to be standard practice; it probably occurs in this setting more than in other health care settings. Prendergast et al [21] found that 48% of patients who die in the ICU have life support withdrawn or withheld, whereas a larger percentage have cardiopulmonary resuscitation (CPR) withheld [21]. Expertise in the decision making about withholding and withdrawing treatments and its clinical application is an essential component of palliative care in the ICU. The decision to withdraw organ systems support must be based on patient preferences and goals, knowledge of the likely outcome of continuing systems support versus withdrawing it, and the risks and benefits of prolonging organ system supportive care. Shared decision-making is the first goal in this process, and is based on communication between physicians, nurses and the patient-family. Decision making can be complicated by the term "life support," which can set unrealistic expectations about what the treatment ultimately will deliver. Some individuals are afraid or reluctant to withdraw life support—even when they are fully aware that ongoing treatment will not achieve survival or quality of life—because stopping "life support" makes them seem or feel as if they are facilitating death or abandoning the patient. Confusion about the ethical and legal basis for withdrawal and withholding of life support persists, particularly in matters of withdrawal of mechanical ventilation. This is reflected in the many studies that describe the wide variability in physician practice about these matters. When presented with patient vignettes and several choices for withdrawal or withholding of CPR, dialysis, or ventilatory support, physicians chose different strategies [22,23]. Studies showed that physicians prefer to withdraw treatments in a particular order, often withdrawing vasopressor agents first and the ventilator last, if at all [24], or they will withhold a therapy, but not withdraw it once instituted [25,26]. Ethical and legal precedents are clear that withholding and withdrawing therapy are ethically equivalent and that the patient's autonomy and right to refuse therapy prevail, even if withdrawal may lead to death [27].

After a decision is made to withdraw ventilatory support, the interdisciplinary team and the family must be prepared. Families should be informed of symptoms that can occur following extubation (dyspnea, anxiety, noisy secretions) and reassured that the means to control symptoms rapidly and aggressively will be at hand. It is critical at this point that the patient, family, and ICU staff understand that the intent of the medication is to control symptoms. Although these medications may induce deep sedation or even contribute to the patient's demise, the principle of "double effect" makes this ethically permissible. Equally important as discussing the symptoms that may occur following ventilator withdrawal, is cautioning the family that demise may not occur immediately following ventilator withdrawal. Patients who have had mechanical ventilation withdrawn have been known to survive hours, days, and even longer. Families often want to know the time from ventilator withdrawal to death; this is highly variable and dependent on clinical situations. Generally, health care providers are poor at predicting this, but families should be given a range of times and be prepared for immediate demise if this is a possibility.

It should be determined if the family wishes to be present during ventilator withdrawal or extubation and what provisions should be made for their support during this time. The patient should be premedicated and sedated before removal of the ventilator and extubation. Opioids are the medication of choice for treatment of dyspnea; benzodiazepines are prescribed for anxiety that inevitably accompanies dyspnea. The ventilator can be withdrawn by two basic methods: direct extubation or "terminal weaning." There is little evidence in the literature to support one technique over another. Some investigators describe a combination of both, with a rapid wean to minimal ventilator settings to allow for appropriate control of symptoms, followed by disconnecting the ventilator, then extubation [28]. Selection of a method should be based on the patient's goals, discomfort, and ability to communicate. If the patient hopes to talk and interact with his family with minimal interference, then extubation is necessary. If the patient is unconscious or airway obstruction threatens the patient's and the family's comfort, ventilator weaning without removal of the endotracheal or tracheostomy tube is preferred. A physician needs to be immediately available with additional opioids and benzodiazepines to assess ongoing symptoms and treat them accordingly. It is critical that symptoms be documented, and assessments of pain or discomfort are noted clearly when opioids are increased. Concerns on the part of nurses and physicians about hastening death with the administration of opioids for dyspnea have not been supported by the literature. Studies that examined the time to death after withdrawal of the ventilator found no difference between those who were medicated for dyspnea and those who were not [29].

Pain and symptom management

Although the traditional imperative of ICU care is to cure, there is an equal obligation to relieve suffering. This is true for all patients, not merely those who are dying. Therapy to resuscitate and support life need not preclude attention to relief of suffering, nor should clinicians be deterred from treating pain aggressively because of fears of destabilizing vital system function. To the contrary, the literature suggests that the physiologic response to unrelieved pain and stress is more deleterious to the critically ill patient from tachycardia and agitation that result in increased myocardial oxygen demand [30,31]. Others studies showed that there are long-term adverse consequences of inadequate pain relief and sedation in critically injured burn patients following prolonged ICU stays. These include a greater incidence of acute stress disorders and posttraumatic stress syndrome [32].

Multiple studies have documented the deficiencies in pain and symptom relief in ICUs. In the SUPPORT Study, more than 60% of families of dying, critically ill patients reported that their loved one had multiple severe symptoms (including pain) in the last 3 days of life [5]. Nelson et al [33] prospectively studied critically ill patients who had cancer who could report their own symptoms. A significant proportion of them experienced pain, anxiety, dyspnea, thirst, and hunger. Severe pain and discomfort have been reported by patients during routine nursing and medical procedures in the ICU, such as suctioning and turning [34,35]. Although the literature reports the barriers and deficiencies in pain and symptom management, there are few evidence-based studies on successful pain management strategies for critically ill patients.

The inability of many patients to self-report their symptoms is a barrier to satisfactory pain management in the ICU. Accurate assessment of pain by nursing staff can be extremely difficult; surveys of patients for retrospective pain reports are fraught with methodologic difficulties. Proxy symptom reports have been studied and validated in patients who had cancer, but in general, health care providers underestimate pain when compared with the patient reports; family proxies do not do much better [36,37]. Reliance on tachycardia, dyspnea, and hypertension as proxies for pain in unconscious patients is not sufficient because there are too many variables that affect these vital signs. Several new assessment tools have been developed, specifically for the noncommunicative patient in the ICU. These rely on vital signs and on nonverbal cues, such as grimacing, splinting, restlessness, and stiffness, with points awarded for these behaviors during rest, turning, or movement [38,39]. With the advent of assessment tools, all pain interventions should be based on repetitive assessments and reassessments for response to therapy. The use of pain medications, solely as needed, is no longer standard of care; parameters that are based on numerical scales should govern titration of medication. The use of protocols for pain management and sedation were shown to decrease ventilator days, decrease the length of stay in the ICU, and diminish the frequency of a pain score that is greater than 2 among patients in the ICU [40,41].

Opioids are the mainstay of pain management in the ICU; continuous intravenous (IV) administration is the preferred approach. Dose titration protocols with guidelines for rescue doses should be implemented. For patients who are dying imminently or who require aggressive palliative care, non-IV routes—with the exception of intramuscular injection—can be considered as a way of minimizing the problems that are associated with IV delivery. Attention should be paid to decreasing as many routine critical care nursing procedures (eg, turning, suctioning, intravenous catheters, blood draws, frequent vital signs) as possible, to minimize the symptoms from these seemingly innocuous activities. Increasing data reveal that significant symptoms are related to these procedures [33], particularly among the dying.

Bereavement and family support

Excellent palliative care in the ICU focuses on the patient and family as the unit of care. It is documented increasingly that families of dying, critically ill patients have extensive psychosocial needs and increased rates of mental and physical illness. More often than not, the patient is incapacitated cognitively and the family—while in a crisis situation and bereaved themselves—must be surrogates for decision making. Good communication is valued by families for emotional support as much as it is valued for information and planning. This may prevent later conflicts and facilitate end-of-life decision-making. The positive impact of hospital-based bereavement services, pastoral care, or family support personnel is becoming increasingly apparent on the long-term psychosocial functioning of surviving families and on other outcomes, such as organ donation [42,43]. They are a vital part of comprehensive palliative care in the ICU setting. Multiple studies showed that the way in which bad news is delivered may have life-long effects on the survivors, grief and bereavement process [44,45]. For all of these reasons, intensive care surgeons and other health care providers should be trained in communication skills, specifically for breaking bad news.

It also is clear that the opportunity to say "good-bye" to loved ones and the degree of satisfaction of how this was accomplished are important correlates with posttraumatic stress disorder during bereavement. Families should have as much opportunity to be with loved ones at the bedside as possible. The opportunity for a family's presence at the bedside of the patient in the ICU is a critical part of successful palliative care. Unrestricted visiting hours in ICUs is becoming the norm; this sociocultural change has gone a long way toward improving the quality of death and dying in ICUs. Studies showed that the presence of family does not affect care adversely, and probably improves it [46]. The presence of family during CPR is more controversial, but data increasingly suggest that this is helpful during bereavement [47]. If families are present, a bereavement counselor, social worker, pastoral care or other specially-trained personnel should be present to support the family, explain procedures, and communicate last wishes and preferences to the health care staff. Despite the high technology environment of the ICU, attention can be paid to the spiritual care and death rituals, as appropriate. Families usually need support in after-death procedures; many have little knowledge of how to navigate the social pathways (eg, funeral homes) following death in the hospital. Social worker or spiritual care worker assistance in these matters should be part of the interdisciplinary care that is provided in the ICU.

Summary

Palliative care for the critically ill has become an increasingly important component of care in the SICU. As the population ages, medical technology continues to offer new treatments that can prolong life, and more and more Americans die in the hospital in critical care settings, the appropriate management of the end-of-life must be part of the clinical expertise of surgeons and intensivists. Part of this expertise must include the components of palliative care (eg, pain and symptom management, psychosocial support, communication skills, shared decision-making) and specialized areas of withdrawal and withholding of life support. Integrating palliative care expertise into the SICU is not straightforward; understanding when and how to make the transition from curative to palliative care can be fraught with uncertainty regarding prognosis and patient preferences. Attention to the principles of good pain management, communication with patient and family, and discussion of goals of care are not just for patients who are at the end-of-life, but are appropriate care for all critically ill patients, regardless of prognosis. In this framework, "intensive care" encompasses palliative and curative care.

References

[1] Knaus WA, Draper EA, Wagner DP, et al. An evaluation of outcome from intensive care in major medical centers. Ann Intern Med 1986;104:410–8.
[2] Chelluri L, Pinsky MR, Donahoe MP, et al. Longterm outcome of critically ill elderly patients requiring intensive care. JAMA 1993;269:3119–23.

[3] Angus DC, Barnato AE, Linde-Zwirble WT, et al. The use of intensive care at the end of life in the United States: an epidemiologic study. Crit Care Med 2004;32:638–43.

[4] Lynn J, Teno JM, Phillips RS, et al. Perceptions by family members of the dying experience of older and seriously ill patients. SUPPORT Investigators. Study to Understand Prognoses and Preferences for Outcomes and Risks of Treatments. Ann Intern Med 1997;126:97–106.

[5] The SUPPORT Investigators. A controlled trial to improve care for the seriously ill and hospitalized patients. JAMA 1995;224:1591–8.

[6] Prendergast T, Luce J. Increasing incidence of withholding and withdrawal of life support from the critically ill. Am J Respir Crit Care Med 1997;155:15–20.

[7] Faber-Langendoen K. A multi-institutional study of care given to patients dying in hospital: ethical and practice implications. Arch Intern Med 1996;156:2130–6.

[8] Knaus WA, Rauss A, Alperovitch A, et al. Do objective estimates of chances for survival influence decision to withhold or withdraw treatment? The French Multicentric Group of ICU Research. Med Decis Making 1990;10:163–71.

[9] Barnato AE, Angus DC. Value and role of intensive care unit outcome prediction models in end-of-life decision making. Crit Care Clin 2004;20:345–62.

[10] Cook D, Rocker G, Marshall J, et al. Withdrawal of mechanical ventilation in anticipation of death in the intensive care unit. N Engl J Med 2003;349:1123–32.

[11] Lilly CM, De Meo DL, Sonna LA, et al. An intensive communication intervention for the critically ill. Am J Med 2000;109:469–75.

[12] Curtis JR. Communicating about end of life care with patients and families in the intensive care unit. Crit Care Clin 2004;20:363–80.

[13] Hickey M. What are the needs of families of critically ill patients? A review of the literature since 1976. Heart Lung 1990;19:401–15.

[14] Lilly CM, Sonna LA, Haley KJ, et al. Intensive communication: four-year follow-up from a clinical practice study. Crit Care Med 2003;31:S394–9.

[15] Schneiderman LJ, Gilmer T, Teetzel HD, et al. Effect of ethics consultations on nonbeneficial life-sustaining treatments in the intensive care setting: a randomized controlled trial. JAMA 2003;290:1166–72.

[16] Murphy PA, Price DM, Stevens M, et al. Under the radar: Ccontributions of the SUPPORT nurses. Nurs Outlook 2001;49:238–42.

[17] Way J, Back AL, Curtis JR. Withdrawing life support and resolution of conflict with families. BMJ 2002;325:1342–5.

[18] Tilden VP, Tolle SW, Garland JM, et al. Decisions about life-sustaining treatment. Impact of physicians' behaviors on the family. Arch Intern Med 1995;155:633–8.

[19] McDonagh JR, Elliott TB, Engelberg RA, et al. Studying communication about end-of-life-care during the ICU family conference: development of a framework. J Crit Care 2002;17:147–60.

[20] Cassell J, Buchman TG, Street S, et al. Surgeons, intensivists and the covenant of care: administrative models and values affecting care at the end of life. Crit Care Med 2003;31:1551–7.

[21] Prendergast T, J Claessens MT, Luce JM. A national survey of end-of-life care for critically ill patients. Am J Respir Crit Care Med 1998;158:1163–7.

[22] Cook DJ, Guyatt GH, Jaeschke R, et al. Determinants in Canadian health care workers of the decision to withdraw life support from the critically ill. JAMA 1995;273:703–8.

[23] Hinshaw DB, Pawlik T, Mosenthal AC, et al. When do we stop, and how do we do it? Medical futility and withdrawal of care. J Am Coll Surg 2003;196:621–49.

[24] Solomon MZ, O'Donnell L, Jenning B, et al. Decisions near the end of life: professional views on life sustaining treatments. Am J Public Health 1993;83(1):14–23.

[25] Asch DA, Christakis NA. Why do some physicians prefer to withdraw some forms of life support over others? Med Care 1996;34:103–11.

[26] Christakis NA, Asch DA. Biases in how physicians choose to withdraw life support. Lancet 1993;342:642–6.

[27] Presidents Commission for the Study of Ethical Problems in Medicine and Biomedical and Behavioral Research. Deciding to forego life-sustaining treatment: a report on the ethical, medical and legal issues in treatment decisions. Washington, DC: US Government Printing Office; 1983.

[28] Rubenfeld GD. Principles and practice of withdrawing life-sustaining treatments. Crit Care Clin 2004;20:435–52.

[29] Wilson WC, Smedira NG, Fink C, et al. Ordering and administration of sedatives and analgesics during the withholding and withdrawal of life support from critically ill patients. JAMA 1992;267:949–53.

[30] Lewis AM, Whipple JK, Michael KA, et al. The effect of analgesic treatment on the physiological consequences of acute pain. Am J Hosp Pharm 1994;51:1539–54.

[31] Epstein J, Breslow MJ. The stress response of critical illness. Crit Care Clin 1999;15:17–33.

[32] Saxe G, Stoddard F, Courney D, et al. Relationship between acute morphine and the course of PTSD in children with burns. J Am Acad Child Adolesc Psychiatry 2001;40:915–21.

[33] Nelson J, Meier D, Oei E, et al. Self-reported symptom experience of critically ill cancer patients receiving intensive care. Crit Care Med 2001;29:277–82.

[34] Puntillo KA. Dimensions of procedural pain and its analgesic management in critically ill surgical patients. Am J Crit Care 1994;3:116–22.

[35] Turner JS, Briggs SJ, Springhorn HE, et al. Patients recollection of intensive care unit experience. Crit Care Med 1990;18:966–8.

[36] Choiniere M, Melzack R, Girard N, et al. Comparisons between patients' and nurses' assessment of pain and medication efficacy in severe burn injuries. Pain 1990;40:143–52.

[37] Desbiens NA, Mueller-Rizner N. How well do surrogates assess the pain of seriously ill patients? Crit Care Med 2000;28:1347–52.

[38] Puntillo KA, Miaskowski C, Kehrle K, et al. Relationship between behavioral and physiological indicators of pain, critical care patients' self-reports of pain and opioid administration. Crit Care Med 1997;25:1159–66.

[39] Puntillo KA, Stannard D, Miaskowski C, et al. Use of a pain assessment and intervention notation (PAIN) tool in critical care nursing practice: nurses evaluations. Heart Lung 2002; 31:303–14.

[40] Kress J, Pohlman AS, O'Connor MF, et al. Daily interruption of sedative infusions in critically ill patients undergoing mechanical ventilation. New Engl J Med 2000;342:1471–7.

[41] Caswell DR, Williams JP, Vallejo M. Improving pain management in critical care. J Qual Improvement 1996;22:702–12.

[42] Iverson K. Grave words: notifying survivors about sudden unexpected deaths. Tucson (AZ): Galen Press; 1999.

[43] Oliver RC, Sturtevant J, Scheetz J, et al. Beneficial effects of a hospital bereavement intervention program after traumatic childhood death. J Trauma 2001;50:440–8.

[44] Linyear AS, Tartaglia A. Family communication coordination: a program to increase organ donation. J Transplant Coord 1999;9:165–74.

[45] Jurkevich GJ, Pierce B, Pananen L, et al. Giving bad news: the family perspective. J Trauma 2000;48:865–73.

[46] Simpson T, Wilson T, Mucken N, et al. Implementation and evaluation of a liberalized visiting policy. Am J Crit Care 1996;5:420–6.

[47] Meyers TA, Eickhard DJ, Guzzzetta C, et al. Family presence during intensive procedures and resuscitation: the experience of family members, nurses and physicians. Am J Nurs 2000; 100:32–42.

ELSEVIER
SAUNDERS

SURGICAL
CLINICS OF
NORTH AMERICA

Surg Clin N Am 85 (2005) 315–328

Surgical Palliative Care in Thoracic Diseases

Steven J. Mentzer, MD

Division of Thoracic Surgery, Department of Surgery, Brigham and Women's Hospital,
Harvard Medical School, 75 Francis Street, Room 259, Boston, MA 02115, USA

Surgery can play an important role in the treatment of patients who have end stage thoracic disease. In nonmalignant lung diseases, lung transplantation can be an option for selected patients. Diseases, such as emphysema, cystic fibrosis, primary pulmonary hypertension, and idiopathic pulmonary fibrosis, can be treated definitively with lung transplantation [1]. Patients who have severe emphysema also may be candidates for lung volume reduction surgery (LVRS). LVRS recently was shown to improve the quality and quantity of life in selected subpopulations of patients who have emphysema [2]. In patients who have malignant disease, surgery can contribute to patient care beyond the initial attempts at curative therapy. For example, it is common for fluid to accumulate in the chest with secondary effects on lung and heart function. In most cases, this fluid accumulation can be effectively treated by palliative surgical interventions.

The dominant symptom that is associated with end stage thoracic disease is dyspnea. Defined as the uncomfortable awareness of breathing, dyspnea is common in patients who have cancer. In a study of a general population of patients who had cancer, 23% of patients reported that their dyspnea was moderate to severe [3]. Patients who had metastatic disease in the thorax were more likely to develop dyspnea [3,4]. Consistent with this finding, 60% of patients who have lung involvement complain of dyspnea. Bruera et al [4], in a study of 135 outpatients at a palliative clinic, found that 74 patients experienced moderate-to-severe dyspnea [4] Nearly three quarters of patients who have advanced cancer report dyspnea in the last 6 weeks of life [5,6].

Surgical palliation of dyspnea focuses on treating effusions of the pleura and pericardium. Pleural effusions are a common complication of malignancy, and malignancy is a common cause of pleural effusions, in general.

E-mail address: smentzer@partners.org

doi:10.1016/j.suc.2004.12.004
surgical.theclinics.com

Malignancy accounts for 20% to 40% of symptomatic pleural effusions [7–9]. Lung cancer, breast cancer, lymphoma, and leukemia account for approximately 75% of all malignancy-associated effusions [8,9]. Congestive heart failure and infection are the other leading causes [8]. Most pericardial effusions that require invasive treatment are the result of malignant disease [10]. In the management of pleural and pericardial effusions, surgical intervention can make a tangible impact on the subjective experience of breathlessness. In many cases, effective surgical therapy of pleural or pericardial effusions also can improve the ability of the patient to perform the routine activities of daily living.

Bilateral pleural effusions

The normal pleural space has approximately 10 mL to 20 mL of fluid with a protein content of 2 g/dL. In normal circumstances, the presumed function of the pleural space, as well as the fluid lubricant, is to facilitate the mechanical coupling between the lung and the surrounding chest wall and diaphragm.

Three pathophysiologic processes that can contribute to the development of pleural effusions: (1) an imbalance in transpleural fluid filtration (passive Starling forces), (2) an impairment of lymphatic drainage, and (3) an increase in mesothelial and capillary endothelial permeability [11]. An imbalance in fluid filtration is the most common cause of bilateral pleural effusions.

Four pressures determine the driving force for fluid filtration rate across a vessel wall: the hydraulic and colloid osmotic pressures in the vessel and the hydraulic and colloid osmotic pressures in the tissue space (Starling forces) [12]. The clinical problems that are associated with an increase in hydraulic pressures include heart failure and hypervolemic states. A pathologic decrease in oncotic pressure can occur in renal failure, hepatic failure, or nutritional deficiencies. The filtration of fluid in excess of reabsorption results in the accumulation of pleural effusions.

An imbalance in fluid filtration can be distinguished from the other two causes of pleural effusions by the protein content of the fluid. Because the filtration occurs across an endothelial barrier, the fluid has a decreased protein content and commonly is referred to as a "transudate." In contrast, the other two causes of pleural effusions typically are associated with relatively increased protein concentrations in the pleural fluid (so-called "exudative" effusions).

Patients who have unexplained bilateral pleural effusions should have a systemic evaluation with particular attention to cardiac, renal, and hepatic function (Fig. 1). A thoracentesis may provide symptomatic benefit and provide an opportunity to assess the protein content in the fluid. A typical patient who has a transudative effusion may have a protein content of

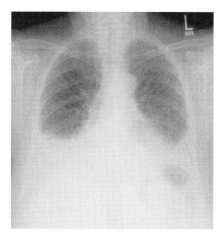

Fig. 1. Bilateral pleural effusions in a patient who has combined congestive failure and hypoproteinemia.

2 g/dL in the effusion and a serum protein content of 6 g/dL. If the protein concentration of the effusion is less than half of the serum concentration, a diagnosis of a transudative effusion is established.

The significance of identifying a transudative effusion is that surgical intervention rarely is beneficial beyond therapeutic thoracentesis. Traditional tube thoracostomy is contraindicated in a patient who has a transudative effusion. Percutaneous tube drainage of bilateral pleural effusions can be hazardous in a patient who has ascites. The placement of a pleural drain in this setting may result in large, ongoing fluid losses that contribute to acute hypovolemia and chronic hypoproteinemia. As an alternative to surgical treatment, appropriate medical therapy should be targeted at the organ dysfunction that is causing the imbalance in fluid filtration.

Unilateral pleural effusion

Unilateral pleural effusions are commonly associated with an impairment of pleural lymphatic drainage or an increase in capillary permeability [11]. Pleural lymphatic drainage is believed to occur through lymphatic stoma. Pleural lymphatic stoma are most prevalent on the anterior chest wall, mediastinal pleura, and along the diaphragmatic pleural surface [13]. These stoma seem to be functionally impaired in the presence of malignancy and in some inflammatory reactions. Frequently coexisting with lymphatic obstruction is the pathologic production of pleural fluid that is caused by an increase in capillary permeability. Most clinically relevant inflammatory reactions are associated with a significant increase in capillary permeability. In addition to inflammation-associated capillary leak, increased permeability has been demonstrated from the intratumoral capillaries [14].

The presence of a pleural effusion is typically detected by chest radiograph (Fig. 2). In most patients who have a continuous pleural space, 150 mL to 200 mL of pleural fluid will cause a blunting of the costophrenic angle in an upright chest radiograph. The primary process that contributes to a unilateral opacity on a chest radiograph may be a pleural effusion or parenchymal lung collapse. Collapsed or atelectatic lung can be distinguished from pleural effusions by an assessment of the volume of the ipsilateral hemithorax. Collapsed lung is associated with tracheal deviation (mediastinal shift), an elevated hemidiaphragm, and decreased intercostal spaces. If there is evidence of a small hemithorax, chest CT scanning is useful to assess the relative contribution of the pleural effusion and atelectatic lung to the opacity that is observed on chest radiograph.

In the setting of a pleural effusion, a diagnostic thoracentesis is indicated. A diagnostic thoracentesis provides insight into: (1) the etiology of the effusion, (2) the size of the effusion, (3) the contribution of the effusion to the patient's symptoms, and (4) the function of the underlying lung. To achieve these goals, the initial diagnostic thoracentesis should remove as much of the fluid as possible. Radiographic heterogeneity or variable echogenicity often is interpreted mistakenly as loculated fluid. Despite the presence of fibrinous septae, most pleural effusions are contiguous fluid collections and can be drained completely by thoracentesis alone.

To help establish the etiology of the effusion, chemical analysis of the fluid can distinguish an exudative pleural effusion from an transudative effusion. The protein content of an exudative effusion typically is greater than 75% of the serum protein concentration. In chronic inflammation,

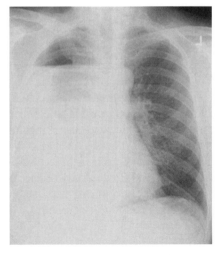

Fig. 2. Unilateral pleural effusion in a patient who has metastatic colon carcinoma. The chest radiograph shows the residual hydropneumothorax from a previous thoracentesis.

such as a *Mycobacterium tuberculosis* infection, the pleural fluid protein concentration may exceed serum concentrations.

In the setting of an unexplained exudative effusion, the most effective diagnostic approach involves thoracentesis and an examination of the cells in the pleural fluid. The diagnostic yield of cytologic examination of pleural fluid cells exceeds 50% in most types of malignant pleural effusion [15]. The yield increases modestly with repeated thoracentesis. Alternatively, the detection of numerous polymorphonuclear leukocytes in the pleural fluid suggests the presence of an inflammatory process. The presence of abundant mononuclear cells can be the most problematic finding. These mononuclear cells may represent normal lymphoid cells in a chronic effusion, reactive cells in a tuberculous infection, or even small cell carcinoma.

The complete evacuation of the pleural fluid provides an assessment of the contribution of the effusion to the patient's dyspnea. With the rapid removal of effusions that are greater than 800 mL, the patient may cough and complain of angina-like chest discomfort. In most cases, these symptoms resolve rapidly with expansion of the lung and normalization of pleural pressures.

The symptomatic benefit of thoracentesis may be delayed because re-expansion of the lung can be associated with regional or "negative pressure" pulmonary edema. Negative pressure pulmonary edema is most commonly seen when thoracentesis is performed ill-advisedly in the setting of a malignant proximal airway obstruction; however, it also may be observed in patients who have functional small airway obstruction (Fig. 3). The simplest physiologic explanation for this observation is that the negative pressure that is applied to the pleural catheter creates a pressure gradient from the alveolar space to the pleural space. Because the transalveolar pressure cannot be equilibrated by air flow, continued expansion of the lung occurs at the expense of fluid accumulation in the lung interstitium. Negative pressure pulmonary edema responds to diuretic therapy and typically resolves within 24 to 48 hours (Fig. 3). Parenchymal edema that

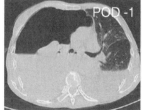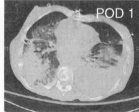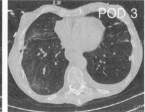

Fig. 3. A patient who has hydropneumothorax that is associated with ovarian carcinoma. The patient had surgical drainage of the hydropneumothorax with significant pulmonary edema on postoperative day (POD) 1. After aggressive diuresis, the pulmonary edema resolved. Note the improvement in the contralateral pleural effusion with diuresis alone (POD 3).

persists for longer than 48 hours may represent infection or lymphangitic tumor.

Lung parenchyma that has been compressed by pleural fluid for weeks to months may not have sufficient compliance to fill the pleural space, despite the removal of the fluid. Postthoracentesis radiographs may show a pneumothorax that is ascribed mistakenly to lung injury during the thoracentesis. The pneumothorax does not reflect acute lung injury, but rather chronic entrapment of the lung . The underlying lung is entrapped, not by a fibrinous peel as seen in pleural empyema, but by remodeling of the underlying lung parenchyma. Although the mechanisms that are involved in lung remodeling are unclear, the process seems to be dependent upon the degree of parenchymal inflammation. Whole-lung atelectasis—occasionally observed in patients who have development-associated tumors—can be reversed completely when the tumor is resected. These cases seem to differ from inflammation- or malignancy-associated pleural effusions in the degree of parenchymal lung inflammation.

The development of indwelling pleural catheters suggests that chronic drainage of the entrapped lung can recruit lung volume. The pleural catheters—similar in design to indwelling Hickman central venous catheters—have a subcutaneous cuff that seals the external portion of the catheter. Typically, the catheter is placed in the operating room to ensure sterility. In most patients, we use general anesthesia and selective lung ventilation for placement of the catheter. A light general anesthetic is used to control patient ventilation and to facilitate bronchoscopy. Bronchoscopy is performed to assess the airway obstruction and for potential secretions. Parenchymal abnormalities can be evaluated with bronchoalveolar lavage cytology and culture.

Selective lung ventilation with a double lumen endotracheal tube also facilitates an assessment of differential lung function. Single-lung ventilation can provide a direct measure of static and dynamic lung compliance. Measuring the fraction of inspired oxygen with the oxygen saturation in the peripheral arterial circulation gives an assessment of gas exchange. Comparing the efficiency of ventilation-perfusion matching in the diseased, as well as the contralateral lung, can be useful in anticipating the patient's subsequent clinical course. For example, in a patient who has a normal contralateral lung, a partially inflated lung with diminished compliance and impaired matching may be disabling. Allowing the diseased lung to become completely atelectatic may decrease the patient's shunt and improve their symptoms.

The visualization of the pleural space is performed using video thoracoscopy. In most cases, a 5-mm thoracoscope is inserted through a 1-cm access port that is placed in the seventh intercostal space in the anterior axillary line. The thoracoscope permits visualization of the visceral and parietal pleural surfaces. Directed biopsies of the pleura can be performed if there is any diagnostic uncertainty. The thoracoscope also can provide visual feedback on the efficacy of lung recruitment maneuvers—typically prolonged end-inspiratory pauses—to increase lung volumes. Lungs that fail to fill a resting (anesthetized) hemithorax, despite maximal positive pressure insufflation, are entrapped. In our experience, patients who have entrapped lungs are unlikely to achieve stable pleural apposition with 24 to 72 hours of negative (-20 to -40 cm H_2O) pleural pressure applied through standard chest tubes.

Patients who have an entrapped lung are more likely to benefit from placement of an indwelling pleural catheter than short-term tube suction. The catheter can be drained intermittently with the use of a properly configured syringe or a proprietary suction bottle. In either case, pleural catheters that are drained several times per week over 6 to 9 weeks can show significant increases in the volume of the underlying lung (Fig. 4). This gradual recruitment of lung volume is potentially useful in facilitating pleural apposition and recruiting lung function. The surface tension that is produced by the simple apposition of visceral and parietal pleura may contribute to limiting the reaccumulation of pleural fluid. In addition, pleural apposition is a prerequisite to any subsequent attempts at mechanical or chemical pleurodesis. The recruitment of lung volume also can be useful in improving the mechanical coupling between the lung and

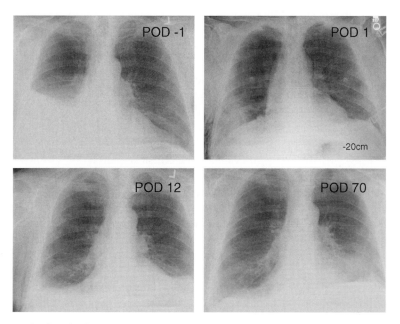

Fig. 4. The chronic effusion was drained by video thoracoscopy on POD 0. On negative pleural pressure (POD 1), the lung was nearly filling the hemithorax. On POD 12, the right basilar effusion returned. Chronic intermittent drainage over the ensuing 8 weeks resulted in near-complete recruitment of the right lung (POD 70).

chest wall and diaphragm, and recruiting alveolar surface area for gas exchange. These potential benefits of lung volume recruitment, however, remain unproven.

In patients who achieve visceral-parietal pleural apposition in the operating room, a surgical option is the fusion of visceral and parietal pleural surfaces to prevent fluid reaccumulation. The procedure that fuses the pleural surfaces is termed a "pleurodesis." Either mechanical or chemical pleurodesis can be performed. Both approaches rely upon inflammation to create a pleural symphysis. Mechanical approaches use abrasives, such as coarse gauze sponges, to denude the pleural mesothelium. In most cases, the usefulness of mechanical pleurodesis tends to be restricted to clinical situations in which localized or focal pleural symphysis is desired.

Chemical pleurodesis has been performed with numerous compounds, including antibiotics, chemotherapeutic agents, and fine-grained minerals. The antibiotics included tetracycline and doxycycline; however, tetracycline is no longer available in the United States in an intravenous form. Both of these antibiotics are associated when intense pleuritic pain when administered in an awake patient. The chemotherapeutic agents include bleomycin and cisplatin. The use of bleomycin, the only agent that is approved by the U.S. Food and Drug Administration for the prevention of recurrent effusions, is limited by its expense. Numerous studies have suggested that all categories of sclerosing agents, including immunotherapy, seem to be similarly effective [16–23]. A meta-analysis of pleurodesis studies reported in 1994, indicated that approximately two thirds of patients responded to pleurodesis and that talc, tetracycline, and bleomycin are comparably effective [9].

Because of cost considerations, talc is the most commonly used agent in the setting of malignancy. Talc is a fine-grained compound that is composed of hydrated magnesium silicate. Sterilized talc can be introduced into the pleural space as a dry powder by insufflation or in a liquid slurry; a comparison of slurry versus powdered talc did not show significant differences [24]. We prefer to evacuate the effusion completely and insufflate dry talc at the time of thoracoscopy. This approach eliminates the uncertain dose effects of bedside talc slurry therapy. Ideally, the talc can be introduced into the pleural space while the patient is spontaneously ventilating under general anesthesia. This results in an even distribution of the talc that can be confirmed by video thoracoscopy. Pleural drainage tubes are placed in the apex and across the diaphragm and are maintained on -20 cm H_2O suction for 48 hours.

Talc and the other sclerosing agents stimulate pleural inflammation that often is associated with pleuritic pain, fever, and hypoxia. The relative hypoxia, which may persist for several days, seems to reflect an inflammation-associated intrapulmonary shunt. The inefficiencies in the treated lung are usually well-tolerated if the patient has a normal contralateral lung. For this reason, bilateral pleurodesis is contraindicated.

Also, caution should be exercised in patients who have significant contralateral parenchymal lung disease. These patients may develop several days of life-threatening hypoxemia that is unresponsive to oxygen therapy. A pleural catheter without active pleurodesis may be a preferable strategy in this group of patients.

The efficacy of talc and the other chemical sclerosing agents seems to be dependent upon pleural apposition, the effective delivery of the sclerosing agent, and adequacy of the inflammatory reaction. Although two thirds of patients seem to have a symptomatic benefit [9], the degree of pleural symphysis is variable. The most reliable pleurodesis occurs laterally and apically, whereas residual fluid is observed commonly across the diaphragm. These observations suggests that pleural movement, particularly the motion of a functioning diaphragm, inhibits pleural symphysis.

Finally, the consequences of pleurodesis on ventilatory function is unknown. One theoretic consideration is that pleurodesis could impair the mechanical coupling of the lung and the chest wall and diaphragm. Support for this concept was observed in a patient who developed progressive respiratory failure after bilateral pleurodesis in the setting of a single functioning diaphragm. In the most cases, however, the impairment of mechanical coupling is likely to be a minor consideration relative to the functional derangements that are caused by the pleural fluid.

Pericardial effusions

Similar pathophysiologic processes are responsible for the accumulation of fluid in the pleura and pericardium. The most significant difference is that most transudative effusions in the pericardium are asymptomatic [25]. Probably because of the adaptive compliance of the pericardium, chronic transudative pericardial effusions can be well-tolerated. In two thirds of patients, the normal amounts of pericardial fluid (10–50 mL) can increase more than 20-fold with no overt cardiac signs or symptoms [25]. In contrast, an impairment of lymphatic drainage or an increase in mesothelial and capillary endothelial permeability often results in more rapid fluid accumulation and a greater incidence of symptomatic pericardial effusions. Dyspnea is the most common initial complaint of patients who have malignant pericardial effusions [26]. The most common malignancies that are associated with pericardial effusions are lung cancer (33%), breast cancer (25%), and lymphoma (15%) [27]. The impairment of heart function as a result of fluid or blood in the pericardial sac is referred to as "tamponade."

The clinical manifestations of pericardial tamponade are dyspnea, tachycardia, and peripheral edema. The components of Beck's triad (hypotension, active jugular veins, diminished heart sounds) usually also are present in patients who have advanced disease. Regardless of the findings on clinical examination, however, the potential diagnosis of pericardial effusion and cardiac tamponade should be considered in patients who have cancer and progressive dyspnea that is out of proportion to the change in their chest radiograph.

The diagnosis of a pericardial effusion can be suggested by chest radiograph (Fig. 5) and established by chest CT scanning or echocardiography. The diagnosis of cardiac tamponade, however, must be established by correlating clinical signs with echocardiographic findings. Two-dimensional echocardiography may show a pericardial effusion, but the diagnosis of cardiac compression may be unclear. Echocardiographic findings of early diastolic collapse of the right ventricular free wall has a specificity of 84% to 100%, but a sensitivity of 38% to 48% [27]. In contrast, late diastolic compression of the right atrium has a sensitivity of 55% and 60% and a specificity of 50% to 68% [27]. A substantial augmentation of right-sided flow with inspiration (Kussmaul sign) also may be noted on echocardiography. Any of these signs is suggestive of clinically significant tamponade [28].

The hemodynamic consequences of the pericardial effusion can be established by percutaneous drainage. Image-guided pericardiocentesis should be performed in all patients who demonstrate evidence of tamponade. Pericardiocentesis confirms the presence of the effusion, provides fluid for diagnostic studies, and decreases the risks of any subsequent general anesthesia. In some cases, pericardiocentesis provides definitive diagnosis and treatment. For example, radiation therapy or chemotherapy can cause pericarditis without malignant involvement of the pericardium. Radiation therapy is usually associated with radiation doses to the pericardium in excess of 30 Gy. This is a dose of radiation that can be

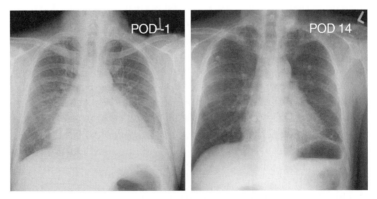

Fig. 5. The pericardial effusion that is suggested by this chest radiograph (POD −1) was confirmed by echocardiography. After a video-assisted pericardotomy, the patient's dyspnea resolved. Note that the spontaneous diuresis after the procedure markedly reduced the patient's associated left pleural effusion (POD 14).

seen in the treatment of lung, esophageal, or breast cancer. In many of these cases, the pericardiocentesis decompresses the pericardium and the inflammation-associated effusion resolves without the need for further intervention.

The reason pericardiocentesis is essential before any surgical intervention is the systemic vasodilatation that is associated with general anesthesia. Because cardiac tamponade restricts normal compensatory mechanisms, general anesthesia can be associated with life-threatening hypotension. All patients who have cardiac dysfunction secondary to a pericardial effusion should have a percutaneous pericardiocentesis performed before general anesthesia and definitive surgical intervention.

Pericardiocentesis is associated with recurrent pericardial effusions in 20% to 50% of patients [29–32]. Patients who have recurrent pericardial effusions should be considered for surgical pericardiotomy. The goal of definitive surgical drainage of a pericardial effusion is to re-establish the lymphatic drainage of the pericardial sac. This can be achieved by creating a communication (or "window") between the pericardium and the pleural space, or the pericardium and adjacent subcutaneous tissues.

The pericardial–pleural window can be performed by video thoracoscopy or anterior thoracotomy [7]. A portion of the pericardium is excised anterior to the phrenic nerve. In situations in which the pericardium is loculated, a second window that is posterior to the phrenic nerve may be indicated. The relative value of drains that are placed in the pericardium at the time of surgery is uncertain. Drains that are placed in the properly decompressed pericardium typically have little output and are removed within 24 to 48 hours.

Because of the common pathophysiology of pleural and pericardial effusions, 50% of patients who have pericardial effusions present with a coexistent pleural effusions (Fig. 6) [7]. Video thoracoscopy of the left

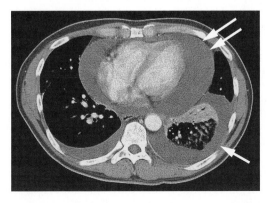

Fig. 6. Combined pericardial (*double arrow*) and pleural (*single arrow*) effusions are observed in half of the patients who have pericardial effusions.

hemithorax provides an opportunity to treat both effusions. The theoretic disadvantage of this approach is that the effusions usually are the consequence of the obstruction of common lymphatics. Because of the diffuse lymphatic disease, the creation of a pericardial–pleural window on the same side as a pleural effusion may not result in reabsorption of the fluid. The benefit of this approach, however, is that the pericardium is decompressed and the secondary effects that are related to cardiac tamponade are improved.

In patients who have limited thoracoscopic access to the pericardium, a subxiphoid pericardial window is an alternative approach. The subxiphoid approach involves a midline incision that extends 4 cm below the xiphoid process. The pericardial window is created by excising 10 cm^2 to 15 cm^2 of anterior pericardium. This approach is believed to have a recurrence rate of approximately 30% in 3 months. The recurrence rates decrease with larger pericardial windows. The smallest recurrence rates are achieved when anterior pericardium is excised from one phrenic nerve to the other phrenic nerve. In addition to removing a larger portion of pericardium, the phrenic nerve-to-phrenic nerve approach also may have the advantage of exposing the pericardial fluid to the lymphatic drainage of both pleural spaces.

In selected patients, the pericardial effusion can be controlled by draining the pericardial space and sclerosing the pericardium. The rationale for this approach is similar to that applied in the pleural space (ie, pericardial effusion should be controlled if there is no space for the fluid to accumulate). Tetracycline has been the most commonly used sclerosing agent for malignant pericardial effusions. Alternative sclerosing agents are identical to those used in pleural disease. Although this approach may be the only option in some patients who have end stage disease, there is a concern that sclerosing the pericardial space may produce a loculated pericardium. In the setting of an incompletely fused pericardium, a recurrent effusion may not be safely accessible by thoracoscopy. This concern is unlikely to be a practical problem if the patient's life expectancy is limited to a few weeks. Pericardial sclerotherapy has been reported to control fluid reaccumulation in 70% to 80% of patients for 30 days [32].

Summary

Most patients who have end stage thoracic disease have moderate to severe dyspnea. The dyspnea may be the result of the underlying lung disease, localized disease progression, or the accumulation of fluid within the chest. The most effectively treated clinical problem at the end of life is secondary fluid accumulation in the pleural space or pericardial sac. Focused surgical intervention can play an important role in treating effusive disease of the pleura and pericardium. Minimally invasive surgical interventions, such as the use of video thoracoscopy, can relieve dyspnea effectively and improve the quality of life for patients who have end stage thoracic disease.

References

[1] Mentzer SJ, Swanson SJ. Lung transplantation. In: Austen KF, Burakoff SJ, Rosen FS, et al, editors. Therapeutic immunology. Malden (MA): Blackwell Science, Inc.; 2001. p. 482–95.
[2] Fishman A, Martinez F, Naunheim K, et al. A randomized trial comparing lung-volume-reduction surgery with medical therapy for severe emphysema. N Engl J Med 2003;348: 2059–73.
[3] Dudgeon DJ, Kristjanson L, Sloan JA, et al. Dyspnea in cancer patients: prevalence and associated factors. J Pain Symptom Manage 2001;21:95–102.
[4] Bruera E, Schmitz B, Pither J, et al. The frequency and correlates of dyspnea in patients with advanced cancer. J Pain Symptom Manage 2000;19:357–62.
[5] Dudgeon DJ, Lertzman M. Dyspnea in the advanced cancer patient. J Pain Symptom Manage 1998;16:212–9.
[6] Reuben DB, Mor V. Dyspnea in terminally ill cancer patients. Chest 1986;89:234–6.
[7] DeCamp MM Jr, Mentzer SJ, Swanson SJ, et al. Malignant effusive disease of the pleura and pericardium. Chest 1997;112:291S–5S.
[8] Marel M, Zrustova M, Stasny B, et al. The incidence of pleural effusion in a well-defined region. Epidemiologic study in central Bohemia. Chest 1993;104:1486–9.
[9] Walker-Renard PB, Vaughan LM, Sahn SA. Chemical pleurodesis for malignant pleural effusions. Ann Intern Med 1994;120:56–64.
[10] Campione A, Cacchiarelli M, Ghiribelli C, et al. Which treatment in pericardial effusion? J Cardiovasc Surg (Torino) 2002;43:735–9.
[11] Zocchi L. Physiology and pathophysiology of pleural fluid turnover. Eur Respir J 2002;20: 1545–58.
[12] Starling EH. On the absorption of fluids from the convective tissue spaces. J Physiol (Lond) 1896;19:312.
[13] Miura T, Shimada T, Tanaka K, et al. Lymphatic drainage of carbon particles injected into the pleural cavity of the monkey, as studied by video-assisted thoracoscopy and electron microscopy. J Thorac Cardiovasc Surg 2000;120:437–47.
[14] Furman-Haran E, Margalit R, Grobgeld D, et al. Dynamic contrast-enhanced magnetic resonance imaging reveals stress-induced angiogenesis in MCF7 human breast tumors. Proc Natl Acad Sci USA 1996;93:6247–51.
[15] Dines DE, Pierre RV, Franzen SJ. The value of cells in the pleural fluid in the differential diagnosis. Mayo Clin Proc 1975;50:571–2.
[16] Emad A, Rezaian GR. Treatment of malignant pleural effusions with a combination of bleomycin and tetracycline. A comparison of bleomycin or tetracycline alone versus a combination of bleomycin and tetracycline. Cancer 1996;78:2498–501.
[17] Gravelyn TR, Michelson MK, Gross BH, et al. Tetracycline pleurodesis for malignant pleural effusions. A 10-year retrospective study. Cancer 1987;59:1973–7.
[18] Heffner JE, Standerfer RJ, Torstveit J, et al. Clinical efficacy of doxycycline for pleurodesis. Chest 1994;105:1743–7.
[19] Martinez-Moragon E, Aparicio J, Rogado MC, et al. Pleurodesis in malignant pleural effusions: a randomized study of tetracycline versus bleomycin. Eur Respir J 1997;10:2380–3.
[20] Nio Y, Nagami H, Tamura K, et al. Multi-institutional randomized clinical study on the comparative effects of intracavital chemotherapy alone versus immunotherapy alone versus immunochemotherapy for malignant effusion. Br J Cancer 1999;80:775–85.
[21] Patz EF Jr, McAdams HP, Erasmus JJ, et al. Sclerotherapy for malignant pleural effusions: a prospective randomized trial of bleomycin vs doxycycline with small-bore catheter drainage. Chest 1998;113:1305–11.

[22] Schafers SJ, Dresler CM. Update on talc, bleomycin, and the tetracyclines in the treatment of malignant pleural effusions. Pharmacotherapy 1995;15:228–35.

[23] Zimmer PW, Hill M, Casey K, et al. Prospective randomized trial of talc slurry vs bleomycin in pleurodesis for symptomatic malignant pleural effusions. Chest 1997;112:430–4.

[24] Yim AP, Chan AT, Lee TW, et al. Thoracoscopic talc insufflation versus talc slurry for symptomatic malignant pleural effusion. Ann Thorac Surg 1996;62:1655–8.

[25] Bisel HF, Wroblewski F, Ladue JS. Incidence and clinical manifestations of cardiac metastases. JAMA 1953;153:712–5.

[26] Warren WH. Malignancies involving the pericardium. Semin Thorac Cardiovasc Surg 2000; 12:119–29.

[27] Chiles C, Woodard PK, Gutierrez FR, et al. Metastatic involvement of the heart and pericardium: CT and MR imaging. Radiographics 2001;21:439–49.

[28] Sagrista-Sauleda J, Merce J, Permanyer-Miralda G, et al. Clinical clues to the causes of large pericardial effusions. Am J Med 2000;109:95–101.

[29] Anderson TM, Ray CW, Nwogu CE, et al. Pericardial catheter sclerosis versus surgical procedures for pericardial effusions in cancer patients. J Cardiovasc Surg (Torino) 2001;42: 415–9.

[30] Celermajer DS, Boyer MJ, Bailey BP, et al. Pericardiocentesis for symptomatic malignant pericardial effusion: a study of 36 patients. Med J Aust 1991;154:19–22.

[31] Girardi LN, Ginsberg RJ, Burt ME. Pericardiocentesis and intrapericardial sclerosis: effective therapy for malignant pericardial effusions. Ann Thorac Surg 1997;64:1422–7.

[32] Martinoni A, Cipolla CM, Civelli M, et al. Intrapericardial treatment of neoplastic pericardial effusions. Herz 2000;25:787–93.

SURGICAL
CLINICS OF
NORTH AMERICA

Surg Clin N Am 85 (2005) 329–345

Surgical and Radiosurgical Management of Brain Metastases

Fred G. Barker II, MD[a,b,]*

[a]*Department of Surgery (Neurosurgery), Harvard Medical School, Boston, MA*
[b]*Brain Tumor Center, Cox 315, Massachusetts General Hospital,*
32 Fruit Street, Boston, MA 02114, USA

Approximately 10% to 15% of all patients who have cancer will be diagnosed with brain metastases in the course of their illness, although the incidence in autopsy studies is greater [1,2]. Most patients live less than a year after diagnosis of brain metastases; however, it probably is the specter of physical and mental disability during that time that is feared most by patients and families. Not all morbidity from brain metastases can be avoided or reversed, but aggressive local treatment is now known to benefit many patients who have one or a few brain metastases. These treatments (surgical resection or focused radiation) are the main subject of this article.

Epidemiology and clinical presentation

Approximately 100,000 to 150,000 patients are diagnosed with brain metastases annually in the United States [1–3]. The most common primary site of origin is lung; melanoma and renal cell and breast carcinoma account for much of the remainder [1]. Common primary histologies for which spread to the brain is uncommon include colorectal, ovarian, and prostate cancer. Presentation with metastasis from a previously unknown primary lesion is common; sometimes, no systemic primary lesion is detected despite extensive imaging. Metastases can be single or, more commonly, multiple (half to two thirds of cases) [2,3]. Most metastases occur at the junction between gray and white matter in the cerebral hemispheres, but deeper supratentorial locations are also common; fewer occur in the cerebellum or

---

* Brain Tumor Center, Cox 315, Massachusetts General Hospital, 32 Fruit Street, Boston, MA 02114.
    E-mail address: barker@helix.mgh.harvard.edu

doi:10.1016/j.suc.2004.11.003   *surgical.theclinics.com*

brain stem [4]. Single brain metastasis refers to one known metastasis in the brain, regardless of systemic status, whereas a solitary brain metastasis is the only known metastatic site. Oligometastatic disease is an arbitrarily defined term, usually implying from one to three or four metastases. Most patients who have brain metastases are diagnosed using contrast-enhanced imaging studies (CT or MRI) (Fig. 1). MRI is the most sensitive study [5].

Symptoms from brain metastases can include headache (the most common symptom), cognitive dysfunction, seizures, or focal neurologic deficits in any combination [2]. Deficits usually develop over days to a few weeks, unless there has been hemorrhage into the lesion—an especially characteristic feature of melanoma and choriocarcinoma metastases. Symptoms of hydrocephalus or gait ataxia from posterior fossa lesions can develop rapidly, even without hemorrhage, and may progress to nausea, vomiting, and obtundation. Focal neurologic deficits usually correspond to the location of at least one of the lesions, although surrounding edema, rather than direct mass effect, causes most symptoms (see Fig. 1).

Medical management

Corticosteroids are administered to symptomatic patients to palliate focal deficits and headache. Symptoms often improve or resolve after a few days of treatment. Aside from rare exceptions (eg, metastases from lymphoma), corticosteroids have no effect on the lesions themselves; if stopped, the symptoms will return unless other treatment has been provided. Patients who have cancer often suffer debilitating long-term side effects from

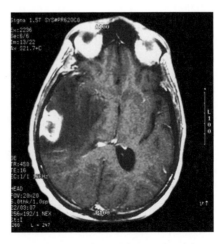

Fig. 1. Axial T1-weighted gadolinium enhanced image of a right temporal brain metastasis from a melanoma primary lesion. The brightly-enhancing metastasis, about 3 cm in size, is surrounded by a 6 cm area of low-signal edema.

prolonged steroid treatment, especially muscle wasting. This presents as difficulty going upstairs or difficulty getting up out of a chair without using the hands; it may not resolve when steroids are stopped. Aseptic necrosis of the femoral heads is a rare, but serious, problem. Prolonged corticosteroid use causes an increased risk of pneumocystis pneumonia; antibacterial prophylaxis is indicated for such patients.

Anticonvulsant prophylaxis against seizures is no longer believed to be beneficial in patients who have brain metastasis, although those who have seizures should be treated [6]. Common anticonvulsants that are metabolized through the hepatic P450 enzyme system (eg, phenytoin, phenobarbital, carbamazepine) can increase metabolism of some common chemotherapy drugs, such as paclitaxel, and cause these agents to reach subtherapeutic blood levels when used at normal dosages [7,8]. When anticonvulsants are necessary for patients who are to receive these agents, valproic acid or levetiracetam (Keppra) may be preferable because these are not P450-inducing drugs.

Methylphenidate (Ritalin) has been tested in patients who had brain metastasis who had neuropsychiatric consequences following whole brain radiotherapy [9,10]. Although favorable results in selected patient cohorts were reported, no randomized trials have been conducted [11].

Most brain metastases respond poorly to systemic chemotherapy [8]. In addition to the usual chemotherapy resistance of solid tumor metastases, the blood–brain barrier can prevent many chemotherapeutics from reaching therapeutic blood levels. For many systemically-administered drugs, like Herceptin (traztuzumab), the central nervous system acts as a sanctuary site; as patients survive longer because of good systemic control, more present with symptomatic brain lesions [12]. Chemotherapy drugs that penetrate the blood-brain barrier, such as temozolomide, are now being tested against brain metastases in phase II trials [13].

Radiotherapy: whole brain treatment

Whole brain fractionated external-beam radiotherapy (WBRT) has been the mainstay of therapy for most patients who have brain metastasis since the 1970s [3,14,15]. WBRT is widely available and produces palliation of symptoms in many patients. Two early Radiation Therapy Oncology Group (RTOG) studies of WBRT plus corticosteroids showed that headaches, impaired cognition, and focal deficits were improved in 35% to 85% of patients; 50% had improved or stable neurologic status for their remaining survival time [14]. More recent studies showed decreased rates of symptomatic improvement (about 30% to 40%), and nearly all patients in poor-prognosis groups remained steroid-dependent [16–18]. The lower response rates in more recent trials may reflect the use of formal patient-based outcome criteria, rather than physician assessments [19]. Median time-to-progression of a single brain metastasis that is treated with WBRT alone is approximately 5 months, and 85% of 1-year survivors have local tumor recurrence [20]. Trials of several radiosensitizers added to WBRT showed negative results [11].

In addition to poor durability of local control, drawbacks of WBRT include short-term toxicities (eg, nausea, fatigue) and frequent long-term steroid dependence. Most patients also lose their hair, although this usually returns in survivors between 6 and 12 months after treatment. Few patients are at risk for long-term radiation toxicity because of short survival (median ~3—4 months after WBRT alone) [14]. Long-term toxicity is usually manifest as leukoencephalopathy on imaging studies (Fig. 2). Symptomatically, neuropsychiatric abnormalities, a syndrome that resembles normal-pressure hydrocephalus (gait ataxia, memory loss, and urinary incontinence), and even frank dementia are seen [21–23]. Although various dose and fractionation schemes that emphasize low fraction size have been tested in an attempt to minimize these potentially devastating effects in patients who have a good prognosis [3], in current practice, WBRT often is omitted when aggressive local therapies (eg, surgery, radiosurgery) are used. As noted below, omitting WBRT inevitably seems to compromise regional control (ie, freedom from new brain metastases).

Radiotherapy: radiosurgery and other highly focused radiation

Radiosurgery is delivery of a single, highly focused, high-dose fraction of radiation using stereotactic targeting techniques, thus achieving high lesion dose with low dose to surrounding normal tissues. Fig. 3 shows a typical

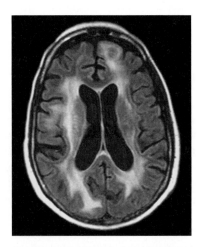

Fig. 2. Axial Fluid Attenuated Inversion Recovery (FLAIR) MRI image of a patient who has leukoencephalopathy due to WBRT. The ventricles are enlarged and are surrounded by bright FLAIR signal indicating widespread damage to deep white matter tracts.

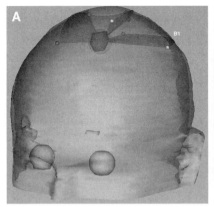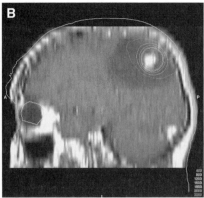

Fig. 3. (*A*) Three-dimensional diagram indicating a single parietal metastasis to be treated using three intersecting arcs of linear accelerator radiation. (*B*) Axial projection showing the lesion surrounded by tightly-spaced isodose contour lines. This reflects the high local dose that is delivered to the lesion while minimizing the dose that is delivered to surrounding normal tissue.

radiosurgery plan for a patient who has a single parietal metastasis. In this example, three intersecting arcs of radiation are delivered using a specially-modified linear accelerator; these intersect at the lesion to produce high dose to the metastasis with little spread into surrounding normal brain tissue (shown by the tightly-spaced isodose lines in Fig. 3B). Radiosurgery can be delivered using a stereotactic head frame or, with some devices, with frameless technique or with a reapplicable head frame for multi-dose (hypofractionated) treatment. Most devices for delivering stereotactic radiosurgery depend on intersection of multiple photon beams to generate the combination of high lesion dose with low normal tissue dose that is characteristic of radiosurgery (see Fig. 3B). It also is possible to exploit the physical characteristics of particle beam radiation (eg, proton beam) to generate a similar dose distribution.

The advantages of radiosurgery are minimal invasiveness and a high degree of durable local tumor control, even for histologies that typically are considered to be radioresistant (eg, melanoma, renal cell carcinoma) [24]. Typically, 1-year actuarial local control of 75% to 85% is reported [25–27]. Higher treatment dosages correlate with better local control; 1-year actuarial local control was 90% for tumors that were treated with doses of 18 Gy or greater compared with 55% for tumors that were treated with 15 Gy to 18 Gy [28]. Treatment of oligometastatic disease is achieved easily in a single treatment session [29,30]; some locations for which surgery is unsuitable (eg, brainstem) are treated easily with radiosurgery [31,32].

Disadvantages of radiosurgery include: (1) limited applicability for large lesions (>3 cm diameter) or for lesions that are too close to critical adjacent structures (eg, optic nerves and chiasm); (2) the length of time (usually several weeks) before tumor shrinkage or reduction of edema is achieved which leads to prolonged steroid treatment in almost half of patients [33]; and (3) the lack of any efficacy against formation of new metastases. Lesions that are larger than 3 cm in diameter or those that are too close to the optic system to be treated safely with radiosurgery sometimes can be treated with hypofractionated radiation using similar targeting techniques and several radiation fractions [34]. Most patients who are treated with radiosurgery have oligometastatic, supratentorial metastases that are minimally symptomatic or for whom a well-tolerated steroid dosage relieves symptoms. Although radiosurgery eventually may palliate symptoms in some patients, its short-term value in this respect is minimal. Of 76 evaluable patients in one trial, only 10 (13%) had improved Karnofsky performance scores after radiosurgery, although 20 of 50 evaluable patients (40%) had improved mental status [35].

Most patients who are treated with radiosurgery also receive immediate WBRT, which increases local control of treated lesions [24,25,36] and regional control (ie, freedom from development of new brain lesions) [24]. In a large, randomized trial of patients who had one to three brain metastases, radiosurgery added to WBRT extended survival by approximately 6 weeks in patients who had one brain metastasis, and improved functional status and reduced steroid dependency in all subgroups [35]. Patients who had two or three metastases did not have a survival benefit from radiosurgery in this trial, despite a benefit that was shown in another smaller randomized trial of patients who had two to four metastases [29]. Some groups defer WBRT after radiosurgery because of the concern of long-term toxicity [37–39]. Radiosurgery, WBRT, or both are then available as salvage treatment for local or regional failure. The merits of this approach are controversial. An ongoing phase III randomized trial is being performed by the American College of Surgeons Oncology Group (www.acosog.org) to compare radiosurgery alone with radiosurgery plus WBRT. The primary end point of the trial is overall survival; important secondary end points include quality of life, duration of independent survival, and freedom from local and regional failure.

Surgical resection

Resection of brain metastases was uncommon before the widespread availability of CT imaging. Since the 1980s, resection of most single brain metastases has become a standard treatment option. Two of three randomized trials that compared resection plus WBRT with WBRT alone that were reported in the 1990s showed increased survival in resected patients [20,40–42]; the annual number of craniotomies in the United States for metastasis resection nearly doubled between 1988 and 2000 [43]. During this time, in-hospital mortality of the procedure decreased from 4.6% to 2.3% and adverse hospital discharge disposition (ie, not directly home) decreased substantially as well [43].

The first benefit of surgery for a brain metastasis is a definitive pathologic diagnosis. With modern imaging techniques, including MRI, the diagnosis of brain metastases usually is secure. Of 127 patients in three randomized trials who had single brain lesions in the context of known systemic cancer, 94% had metastases on histologic confirmation; the remaining patients had gliomas (3%), abscesses (2%), or nonspecific inflammatory lesions (1%) [20,40–42]. Uncertainty may arise, however, particularly when a single brain lesion is seen on MRI without a known history of active systemic cancer. Although resection often is indicated for these patients for diagnosis and treatment, in the unusual situation in which a definitive diagnosis is necessary to guide treatment but resection is not indicated, a stereotactic needle biopsy can be performed. This procedure requires only a short hospital stay (overnight or outpatient); has low morbidity; and in combination with modern immunohistochemical techniques, often can suggest the location of the primary tumor when body imaging is negative. Brain abscesses usually are diagnosed accurately on MRI because of the availability of diffusion-weighted imaging on which abscesses typically are bright and metastases are dark (Fig. 4). Needle biopsy of many abscesses is necessary to guide antibiotic treatment.

Many retrospective case series that were published in the 1980s suggested a survival benefit from resection of single brain metastases; however, the possibility that selection bias might explain the results remained. The first randomized trial of resection of single brain metastases was published in 1990 [20]. Median survival was 40 weeks in resected patients compared with 15 weeks in controls. Freedom from death due to neurologic causes and duration of functional independence also were significantly longer in resected patients. A second randomized trial, first reported in 1993, had

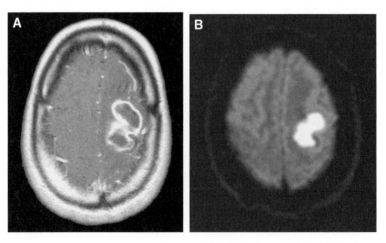

Fig. 4. Brain abscess. Although the axial T1-weighted MRI (*A*) could be consistent with a cystic metastasis, the bright signal on diffusion-weighted MRI (*B*) is characteristic of abscess.

similar results; survival benefit in this trial was limited to patients who had inactive extracranial disease [41,42]. Functional independence was longer, but not significantly so, in resected patients in this trial. The third randomized trial found no extension of survival with resection. In this trial, most patients had active extracranial disease with metastases and poor performance scores; almost half of the patients who received radiation alone underwent surgery after randomization because of patient choice or symptomatic deterioration [40].

Symptomatic improvement is common after surgical removal of a metastasis; it often is apparent in the immediate postoperative period and usually begins by a few days postoperatively at the latest (after the period of postoperative swelling, usually worst 2 to 3 days after operation). Tan and Black [44] reported that 70% of symptomatic patients had resolution of symptoms, 14% were improved, 12% were unchanged, and 4% were worse. Median length of hospital stay was 3 days. Similar results have been reported by other groups [45].

After resection of a metastasis, WBRT is prescribed commonly to prevent local and regional recurrence. A randomized trial that was reported in 1998 supports this practice [46]. Recurrence anywhere in the brain occurred in 18% of radiated patients in this trial compared with 70% of controls. Radiated patients had decreased rates of local (resected lesion) and regional recurrence. Survival and independent survival, however, were not significantly different between the groups. Some centers offer a stereotactic radiosurgery treatment to the resection bed in patients who have undergone single metastasis resection. Trials of some surgically implanted therapies to improve local control without WBRT (eg, permanent low-dose brachytherapy implants or chemotherapy-impregnated polymer wafers) are ongoing.

Of patients who have single brain metastases, about half are poor candidates for surgery because of inaccessibility of the lesion or systemic illness. Assuming that two thirds of patients who have brain metastasis have multiple lesions, and estimating the total annual number of new cases of brain metastasis in the Unites States conservatively at 100,000, roughly 16,500 patients would be expected to undergo resection annually in the United States. Only approximately 7000 such procedures were performed in the United States in 2000; this indicates that this treatment may be underused in current U.S. medical practice [43].

Surgery for multiple or recurrent metastases

The single metastasis is the indication for which the best information favors surgical treatment; resection is performed as the initial therapy. Surgery also can be useful in selected patients who do not conform to this narrow indication. Results of resection of multiple metastases were reported in 1993 by Bindal et al [45]. When all lesions were resected, median survival was 14 months, similar to that for a group of patients who had resection of single metastases at the same institution. Symptomatic improvement was seen in 83% of patients, again similar to results after resection of single metastases. In contrast, patients in whom not all lesions were resected had shorter survival (median 5 months) and only 65% had improvement in symptoms. In current practice, patients who have multiple metastases probably more often undergo resection of a single symptomatic lesion and radiation treatment of the remaining lesions [44]. This strategy also can provide good results, especially in oligometastatic disease when all lesions are treated with surgery or radiosurgery [47]. Aggressive treatment of multiple brain metastases is most appropriate for patients who have oligometastatic brain disease who have good functional status and in whom extracranial disease is well-controlled.

Even when patients have undergone aggressive treatment of a single brain metastasis, some still die from uncontrolled recurrent intracranial disease. When extracranial disease is well-controlled and functional status is good, patients who have intracranial metastases that recur after surgery or radiosurgery may benefit from resection of the recurrent lesion. Arbit et al [48] reported a median survival of 10 months from the time of second operation in 32 patients who had nonsmall cell lung cancer who underwent such resections; similar results were reported in a group of patients who had mixed primary histology [49]. In current practice, patients with recurrent metastases after surgery might be treated with radiosurgery if the lesions were minimally symptomatic and suitable in size and location. When lesions that recur after surgery or radiosurgery with WBRT are resected, some surgeons implant low-activity permanent brachytherapy seeds to prevent a second local recurrence. Bindal et al [49] reported resection of second and third recurrences (ie, a third or fourth craniotomy) with good results; however, this probably reflects selection bias in addition to the effects of resection itself.

Surgery versus radiosurgery

It is clear that surgical resection and stereotactic radiosurgery offer good results for selected patients who have oligometastatic brain disease; many patients are eligible for either of the two treatments. Neither treatment has displaced the other from the standard armamentarium. Despite frequent calls for a randomized study to compare the two treatments, no study has been performed; patient and physician bias are likely to pose significant obstacles to the performance of such a study in the near future.

Several nonrandomized comparisons between resection and radiosurgery for single metastases have been reported [50–52]. Although some studies found longer survival after surgical resection [53], most have found essentially identical survival results after the two treatments [51,52,54]. This is not surprising because treatment mortality is low for both procedures, and most later deaths result from extracranial disease progression. A major drawback of these studies has been the lack of comparisons based on quality of life or resolution of symptoms after treatment. Such information is difficult to acquire retrospectively; a prospective comparison of the two treatments in these respects would be a major contribution to the available evidence. In the absence of such data, cost comparisons of surgery and radiosurgery are of little value, particularly because the available studies fail to adjust for differences between patients who underwent either procedure with respect to symptomatic status, method of diagnosis (patients who undergo surgery frequently are admitted through the emergency ward for treatment of symptoms and systemic work-up before operation, whereas radiosurgery normally is an elective outpatient procedure), and other important differences between patient populations [55–58].

In practical terms, when used as treatment for single brain metastases, radiosurgery and surgical resection offer similar success rates with respect to patient survival. Differences in local control rates between the two treatments may favor radiosurgery, but given the availability of radio-surgery as effective salvage treatment after postsurgical recurrence, this probably is not an important end point for most patients. Surgery probably provides resolution of symptoms from metastases more quickly and more reliably than radiosurgery, although formal comparisons are lacking. Surgery, therefore, seems to be the preferred treatment for accessible metastases with significant symptoms, whereas radiosurgery is preferred for less symptomatic lesions or for lesions for which surgical morbidity would be prohibitive. Because even minor swelling after radiosurgery can cause hydrocephalus when the treated lesion is in the posterior fossa, surgeons often recommend resection of cerebellar metastases, except for smaller lesions. Multiple, minimally symptomatic metastases are treated more simply with radiosurgery unless all are accessible through a single craniotomy. When one of several metastases is symptomatic, resection of that lesion and radiosurgery for the remaining ones may be best.

Metastases from specific primary tumors

Lung cancer is the most common origin for brain metastases; eventually, approximately 20% of patients are affected [1]. In nonsmall cell cancer, metastases most often occur within a short time of diagnosis—typically less than 1 year [59]. A significant proportion of patients present with "synchronous" metastases (ie, metastases present at the time of diagnosis of the chest tumor). When there is only one brain metastasis and no systemic or lymph node metastases, some groups advocate attempted resection of the brain metastasis and the lung mass [60,61]. Because the risk of brain metastasis development is high in locally advanced stage III nonsmall cell lung cancer [62], some groups have investigated the role of prophylactic cerebral irradiation (PCI) in patients who are to undergo intensive treatment for their chest disease [63,64]. Although early results have been promising, further testing in clinical trials is necessary. In small cell lung cancer (SCLC), approximately 10% of patients present with brain metastases and nearly half of the remainder will develop brain metastases during the course of their disease [65]. Metastases from SCLC typically are multiple and grow rapidly. PCI that was administered to patients who were in complete remission after initial SCLC treatment systematic extended survival and disease-free survival in reviews of randomized trials [66,67]. For patients who develop SCLC metastases to the brain, WBRT is the mainstay of treatment. When PCI has been given already, radiation options are limited; chemotherapy plus local treatment (surgery or radiosurgery) for symptomatic lesions usually is chosen.

Breast cancer metastases often occur many years after diagnosis of the primary lesion; approximately 5% of patients are affected [59,68]. Brain metastases are more common in younger patients who have breast cancer [1,59]. Occasionally, they may be extra-axial (dural-based) and mimic meningioma. When a single, small, dural-based mass is found in a patient who has breast cancer and no other metastases, the diagnostic distinction becomes an important one. Negative estrogen receptor status is a risk factor for brain metastasis development; the status of HER2 overexpression is not clear [69]. Brain metastases are uncommon as the only site of metastatic involvement and usually are accompanied by systemic metastases. Aggressive treatment of the brain disease with resection or radiosurgery often is warranted because many systemic metastases are chemosensitive and lengthy survival is not unusual [70].

Colorectal carcinoma causes brain metastases infrequently and affects only approximately 2% of patients [1,59]. Metastases may be cystic; the posterior fossa location is not uncommon and is associated with poor survival [71]. Metastases from esophageal carcinoma, once rare, are becoming increasingly common as survival from locally advanced disease improves [72]. Cystic lesions are common and can progress rapidly; resection may be preferred in these cases.

Renal cell carcinoma spreads to the brain in approximately 5% to 10% of patients, usually 2 to 3 years after diagnosis of the primary lesion, but sometimes not until many years later [1,59,73]. In patients who have renal cell cancer with a mass or masses in the posterior fossa, von Hippel-Lindau syndrome (which causes cerebellar hemangioblastomas) must be considered. Renal cell metastases to the brain, as elsewhere in the body, can be vascular; however, this does not prevent successful resection [74]. Radiosurgery also is effective [24,75].

Melanoma metastases present with overt hemorrhage or microhemorrhage (demonstrated on magnetic resonance susceptibility sequences) more frequently than any other histologic type of metastasis. Approximately 7% of patients who have melanoma—often those who have known regional or distant spread—will develop brain metastases [1]. Typically, brain metastases occur several years after diagnosis of the primary lesion [76,77]. Despite a reputation for radioresistance, brain metastases from melanoma respond well to radiosurgery [24,78,79]. Chemotherapy with temozolomide, an oral alkylating agent that penetrates the blood–brain barrier, also is being investigated [13,80].

Prostate carcinoma, despite its frequency in the population, is a rare source of brain metastases. Nearly all patients have systemically advanced disease [81]. There is a slight predilection for the cerebellum. Surgery and radiosurgery have been used [81]. Ovarian carcinoma spreads to the brain in less than 1% of patients, often as the only metastatic site [82]. Median time between diagnosis of primary lesion and metastasis is approximately 2 years [83]. Surgery and radiosurgery are options [83,84].

Metastases from unknown primary tumors, despite adequate systemic imaging evaluations, usually are diagnosed surgically [85]. When a primary cancer can be identified, lung is the most common histology [86,87]. The absence of extracranial disease is associated with prolonged survival [87]. Radiosurgery also has been used in these patients [88].

Summary

When should surgery be used? First, when there is a need to establish the diagnosis of metastatic cancer, particularly in patients who have no known primary lesion. Second, as an effective therapy in patients who have a single brain metastasis, symptomatic or recurrent metastases, or when a metastasis threatens hydrocephalus if treated with radiation alone. Surgery is probably more effective in relieving symptoms from metastases than other treatments, although formal proof of this is lacking. Stereotactic radiosurgery can replace resection when the metastases are smaller than 3 cm and symptoms can be controlled with an acceptable steroid dose. Location of larger lesions in the posterior fossa is a relative contraindication to radiosurgery. The best candidates for resection and radiosurgery are those who have good systemic control of the primary disease; older age is a relative contraindication to resection. Aggressive treatment of oligometastatic brain disease probably is underused in current U.S. practice.

References

[1] Barnholtz-Sloan JS, Sloan AE, Davis FG, et al. Incidence proportions of brain metastases in patients diagnosed (1973 to 2001) in the Metropolitan Detroit Cancer Surveillance System. J Clin Oncol 2004;22(14):2865–72.
[2] Patchell RA. Brain metastases. In: Black PM, Loeffler J, editors. Cancer of the nervous system. Cambridge (MA): Blackwell Science; 1997. p. 653–63.

[3] Sneed PK. Metastatic brain tumors. In: Prados MD, editor. Brain cancer. Hamilton (Ontario): BC Decker; 2002. p. 375–90.

[4] Delattre JY, Krol G, Thaler HT, et al. Distribution of brain metastases. Arch Neurol 1988; 45:741–4.

[5] Yokoi K, Kamiya N, Matsuguma H, et al. Detection of brain metastasis in potentially operable non-small cell lung cancer: a comparison of CT and MRI. Chest 1999;115(3): 714–9.

[6] Glantz MJ, Cole BF, Forsyth PA, et al. Practice parameter: anticonvulsant prophylaxis in patients with newly diagnosed brain tumors. Report of the Quality Standards Subcommittee of the American Academy of Neurology. Neurology 2000;54(10):1886–93.

[7] Fetell MR, Grossman SA, Fisher JD, et al. Preirradiation paclitaxel in glioblastoma multiforme: efficacy, pharmacology, and drug interactions. New Approaches to Brain Tumor Therapy Central Nervous System Consortium. J Clin Oncol 1997;15(9):3121–8.

[8] van den Bent MJ. The role of chemotherapy in brain metastases. Eur J Cancer 2003;39(15): 2114–20.

[9] Meyers CA, Weitzner MA, Valentine AD, et al. Methylphenidate therapy improves cognition, mood, and function of brain tumor patients. J Clin Oncol 1998;16(7):2522–7.

[10] DeLong R, Friedman H, Friedman N, et al. Methylphenidate in neuropsychological sequelae of radiotherapy and chemotherapy of childhood brain tumors and leukemia. J Child Neurol 1992;7(4):462–3.

[11] Tsao MN, Sultanem K, Chiu D, et al. Supportive care management of brain metastases: what is known and what we need to know. Conference proceedings of the National Cancer Institute of Canada (NCIC) Workshop on Symptom Control in Radiation Oncology. Clin Oncol (R Coll Radiol) 2003;15(7):429–34.

[12] Bendell JC, Domchek SM, Burstein HJ, et al. Central nervous system metastases in women who receive trastuzumab-based therapy for metastatic breast carcinoma. Cancer 2003; 97(12):2972–7.

[13] Agarwala SS, Kirkwood JM, Gore M, et al. Temozolomide for the treatment of brain metastases associated with metastatic melanoma: a phase II study. J Clin Oncol 2004;22(11): 2101–7.

[14] Borgelt B, Gelber R, Kramer S, et al. The palliation of brain metastases: final results of the first two studies by the Radiation Therapy Oncology Group. Int J Radiat Oncol Biol Phys 1980;6(1):1–9.

[15] Gelber RD, Larson M, Borgelt BB, et al. Equivalence of radiation schedules for the palliative treatment of brain metastases in patients with favorable prognosis. Cancer 1981;48(8): 1749–53.

[16] Gerrard GE, Prestwich RJ, Edwards A, et al. Investigating the palliative efficacy of whole-brain radiotherapy for patients with multiple-brain metastases and poor prognostic features. Clin Oncol (R Coll Radiol) 2003;15(7):422–8.

[17] Bezjak A, Adam J, Barton R, et al. Symptom response after palliative radiotherapy for patients with brain metastases. Eur J Cancer 2002;38(4):487–96.

[18] Bezjak A, Adam J, Panzarella T, et al. Radiotherapy for brain metastases: defining palliative response. Radiother Oncol 2001;61(1):71–6.

[19] Hoskin PJ. Case selection in the management of cerebral metastases. Clin Oncol (R Coll Radiol) 2003;15(7):420–1.

[20] Patchell RA, Tibbs PA, Walsh JW, et al. A randomized trial of surgery in the treatment of single metastases to the brain. N Engl J Med 1990;322(8):494–500.

[21] DeAngelis LM, Delattre JY, Posner JB. Radiation-induced dementia in patients cured of brain metastases. Neurology 1989;39(6):789–96.

[22] Sundaresan N, Galicich JH, Deck MDF, et al. Radiation necrosis after treatment of solitary intracranial metastases. Neurosurgery 1981;8:329–33.

[23] Asai A, Matsutani M, Kohno T, et al. Subacute brain atrophy after radiation therapy for malignant brain tumor. Cancer 1989;63(10):1962–74.

[24] Brown PD, Brown CA, Pollock BE, et al. Stereotactic radiosurgery for patients with "radioresistant" brain metastases. Neurosurgery 2002;51(3):656–65 [discussion 665–7].

[25] Flickinger JC, Kondziolka D, Lunsford LD, et al. A multi-institutional experience with stereotactic radiosurgery for solitary brain metastasis. Int J Radiat Oncol Biol Phys 1994; 28(4):797–802.

[26] Shu HKG, Sneed PK, Shiau CY, et al. Factors influencing survival after gamma knife radiosurgery for patients with single and multiple brain metastases. Cancer J Sci Am 1996; 2(6):335.

[27] Loeffler JS, Barker FG, Chapman PH. Role of radiosurgery in the management of central nervous system metastases. Cancer Chemother Pharmacol 1999;43(Suppl):S11–4.

[28] Shiau CY, Sneed PK, Shu HK, et al. Radiosurgery for brain metastases: relationship of dose and pattern of enhancement to local control. Int J Radiat Oncol Biol Phys 1997;37(2): 375–83.

[29] Kondziolka D, Patel A, Lunsford LD, et al. Stereotactic radiosurgery plus whole brain radiotherapy versus radiotherapy alone for patients with multiple brain metastases. Int J Radiat Oncol Biol Phys 1999;45(2):427–34.

[30] Suzuki S, Omagari J, Nishio S, et al. Gamma knife radiosurgery for simultaneous multiple metastatic brain tumors. J Neurosurg 2000;93(Suppl 3):30–1.

[31] Huang CF, Kondziolka D, Flickinger JC, et al. Stereotactic radiosurgery for brainstem metastases. J Neurosurg 1999;91(4):563–8.

[32] Shuto T, Fujino H, Asada H, et al. Gamma knife radiosurgery for metastatic tumours in the brain stem. Acta Neurochir (Wien) 2003;145(9):755–60.

[33] Shaw E, Scott C, Souhami L, et al. Radiosurgery for the treatment of previously irradiated recurrent primary brain tumors and brain metastases: initial report of radiation therapy oncology group protocol (90–05). Int J Radiat Oncol Biol Phys 1996;34(3):647–54.

[34] Manning MA, Cardinale RM, Benedict SH, et al. Hypofractionated stereotactic radiotherapy as an alternative to radiosurgery for the treatment of patients with brain metastases. Int J Radiat Oncol Biol Phys 2000;47(3):603–8.

[35] Andrews DW, Scott CB, Sperduto PW, et al. Whole brain radiation therapy with or without stereotactic radiosurgery boost for patients with one to three brain metastases: phase III results of the RTOG 9508 randomised trial. Lancet 2004;363(9422):1665–72.

[36] Chidel MA, Suh JH, Reddy CA, et al. Application of recursive partitioning analysis and evaluation of the use of whole brain radiation among patients treated with stereotactic radiosurgery for newly diagnosed brain metastases. Int J Radiat Oncol Biol Phys 2000;47(4): 993–9.

[37] Sneed PK, Lamborn KR, Forstner JM, et al. Radiosurgery for brain metastases: is whole brain radiotherapy necessary? Int J Radiat Oncol Biol Phys 1999;43(3):549–58.

[38] Sneed PK, Suh JH, Goetsch SJ, et al. A multi-institutional review of radiosurgery alone vs. radiosurgery with whole brain radiotherapy as the initial management of brain metastases. Int J Radiat Oncol Biol Phys 2002;53(3):519–26.

[39] Hasegawa T, Kondziolka D, Flickinger JC, et al. Brain metastases treated with radiosurgery alone: an alternative to whole brain radiotherapy? Neurosurgery 2003;52(6):1318–26 [discussion 1326].

[40] Mintz AH, Kestle J, Rathbone MP, et al. A randomized trial to assess the efficacy of surgery in addition to radiotherapy in patients with a single cerebral metastasis. Cancer 1996;78(7): 1470–6.

[41] Vecht CJ, Haaxma-Reiche H, Noordijk EM, et al. Treatment of single brain metastasis: radiotherapy alone or combined with neurosurgery? Ann Neurol 1993;33(6):583–90.

[42] Noordijk EM, Vecht CJ, Haaxma-Reiche H, et al. The choice of treatment of single brain metastasis should be based on extracranial tumor activity and age. Int J Radiat Oncol Biol Phys 1994;29(4):711–7.

[43] Barker FG II. Craniotomy for the resection of metastatic brain tumors in the US, 1988–2000. Cancer 2004;100(5):999–1007.

[44] Tan TC, Black PMCL. Image-guided craniotomy for cerebral metastases: techniques and outcomes. Neurosurgery 2003;53(1):82–9 [discussion 89–90].

[45] Bindal RK, Sawaya R, Leavens ME, et al. Surgical treatment of multiple brain metastases. J Neurosurg 1993;79(2):210–6.

[46] Patchell RA, Tibbs PA, Regine WF, et al. Postoperative radiotherapy in the treatment of single metastases to the brain: a randomized trial. JAMA 1998;280(17):1485–9.

[47] Pollock BE, Brown PD, Foote RL, et al. Properly selected patients with multiple brain metastases may benefit from aggressive treatment of their intracranial disease. J Neurooncol 2003;61(1):73–80.

[48] Arbit E, Wronski M, Burt M, et al. The treatment of patients with recurrent brain metastases. A retrospective analysis of 109 patients with nonsmall cell lung cancer. Cancer 1995;76(5):765–73.

[49] Bindal RK, Sawaya R, Leavens ME, et al. Reoperation for recurrent metastatic brain tumors. J Neurosurg 1995;83(4):600–4.

[50] Pollock BE, Brown PD. Stereotactic radiosurgery for brain metastases. In: Pollock BE, editor. Contemporary stereotactic radiosurgery: technique and evaluation. Armonk (NY): Futura; 2002. p. 245–61.

[51] O'Neill BP, Iturria NJ, Link MJ, et al. A comparison of surgical resection and stereotactic radiosurgery in the treatment of solitary brain metastasis. Int J Radiat Oncol Biol Phys 2003; 55(5):1169–76.

[52] Schoggl A, Kitz K, Reddy M, et al. Defining the role of stereotactic radiosurgery versus microsurgery in the treatment of single brain metastases. Acta Neurochir (Wien) 2000; 142(6):621–6.

[53] Bindal AK, Bindal RK, Hess KR, et al. Surgery versus radiosurgery in the treatment of brain metastasis. J Neurosurg 1996;84(5):748–54.

[54] Muacevic A, Kreth FW, Horstmann GA, et al. Surgery and radiotherapy compared with gamma knife radiosurgery in the treatment of solitary cerebral metastases of small diameter. J Neurosurg 1999;91(1):35–43.

[55] Mehta M, Noyes W, Craig B, et al. A cost-effectiveness and cost-utility analysis of radiosurgery vs. resection for single-brain metastases. Int J Radiat Oncol Biol Phys 1997; 39(2):445–54.

[56] Rutigliano MJ, Lunsford LD, Kondziolka D, et al. The cost effectiveness of stereotactic radiosurgery versus surgical resection in the treatment of solitary metastatic brain tumors. Neurosurgery 1995;37(3):445–53 [discussion 453–5].

[57] Wellis G, Nagel R, Vollmar C, et al. Direct costs of microsurgical management of radiosurgically amenable intracranial pathology in Germany: an analysis of meningiomas, acoustic neuromas, metastases and arteriovenous malformations of less than 3 cm in diameter. Acta Neurochir (Wien) 2003;145(4):249–55.

[58] Ott K. A comparison of craniotomy and Gamma Knife charges in a community-based Gamma Knife Center. Stereotact Funct Neurosurg 1996;66(Suppl 1):357–64.

[59] Schouten LJ, Rutten J, Huveneers HA, et al. Incidence of brain metastases in a cohort of patients with carcinoma of the breast, colon, kidney, and lung and melanoma. Cancer 2002; 94(10):2698–705.

[60] Billing PS, Miller DL, Allen MS, et al. Surgical treatment of primary lung cancer with synchronous brain metastases. J Thorac Cardiovasc Surg 2001;122(3):548–53.

[61] Bonnette P, Puyo P, Gabriel C, et al. Surgical management of non-small cell lung cancer with synchronous brain metastases. Chest 2001;119(5):1469–75.

[62] Ceresoli GL, Reni M, Chiesa G, et al. Brain metastases in locally advanced nonsmall cell lung carcinoma after multimodality treatment: risk factors analysis. Cancer 2002;95(3): 605–12.

[63] Stuschke M, Eberhardt W, Pottgen C, et al. Prophylactic cranial irradiation in locally advanced non-small-cell lung cancer after multimodality treatment: long-term follow-up and investigations of late neuropsychologic effects. J Clin Oncol 1999;17(9):2700–9.

[64] Pottgen C, Eberhardt W, Stuschke M. Prophylactic cranial irradiation in lung cancer. Curr Treat Options Oncol 2004;5(1):43–50.

[65] Quan AL, Videtic GM, Suh JH. Brain metastases in small cell lung cancer. Oncology (Huntingt) 2004;18(8):961–72.

[66] Meert AP, Paesmans M, Berghmans T, et al. Prophylactic cranial irradiation in small cell lung cancer: a systematic review of the literature with meta-analysis. BMC Cancer 2001;1(1):5.

[67] Auperin A, Arriagada R, Pignon JP, et al. Prophylactic cranial irradiation for patients with small-cell lung cancer in complete remission. Prophylactic Cranial Irradiation Overview Collaborative Group. N Engl J Med 1999;341(7):476–84.

[68] Chang EL, Lo S. Diagnosis and management of central nervous system metastases from breast cancer. Oncologist 2003;8(5):398–410.

[69] Lin NU, Bellon JR, Winer EP. CNS metastases in breast cancer. J Clin Oncol 2004;22(17):3608–17.

[70] Wronski M, Arbit E, McCormick B. Surgical treatment of 70 patients with brain metastases from breast carcinoma. Cancer 1997;80(9):1746–54.

[71] Wronski M, Arbit E. Resection of brain metastases from colorectal carcinoma in 73 patients. Cancer 1999;85(8):1677–85.

[72] Weinberg JS, Suki D, Hanbali F, et al. Metastasis of esophageal carcinoma to the brain. Cancer 2003;98(9):1925–33.

[73] Cimatti M, Salvati M, Caroli E, et al. Extremely delayed cerebral metastasis from renal carcinoma: report of four cases and critical analysis of the literature. Tumori 2004;90(3):342–4.

[74] Wronski M, Arbit E, Russo P, et al. Surgical resection of brain metastases from renal cell carcinoma in 50 patients. Urology 1996;47(2):187–93.

[75] Sheehan JP, Sun MH, Kondziolka D, et al. Radiosurgery in patients with renal cell carcinoma metastasis to the brain: long-term outcomes and prognostic factors influencing survival and local tumor control. J Neurosurg 2003;98(2):342–9.

[76] Fife KM, Colman MH, Stevens GN, et al. Determinants of outcome in melanoma patients with cerebral metastases. J Clin Oncol 2004;22(7):1293–300.

[77] Sampson JH, Carter JH Jr, Friedman AH, et al. Demographics, prognosis, and therapy in 702 patients with brain metastases from malignant melanoma. J Neurosurg 1998;88(1):11–20.

[78] Seung SK, Sneed PK, McDermott MW, et al. Gamma knife radiosurgery for malignant melanoma brain metastases. Cancer J Sci Am 1998;4(2):103–9.

[79] Mori Y, Kondziolka D, Flickinger JC, et al. Stereotactic radiosurgery for cerebral metastatic melanoma: factors affecting local disease control and survival. Int J Radiat Oncol Biol Phys 1998;42(3):581–9.

[80] Bafaloukos D, Tsoutsos D, Fountzilas G, et al. The effect of temozolomide-based chemotherapy in patients with cerebral metastases from melanoma. Melanoma Res 2004;14(4):289–94.

[81] Tremont-Lukats IW, Bobustuc G, Lagos GK, et al. Brain metastasis from prostate carcinoma: The M. D. Anderson Cancer Center experience. Cancer 2003;98(2):363–8.

[82] Cohen ZR, Suki D, Weinberg JS, et al. Brain metastases in patients with ovarian carcinoma: prognostic factors and outcome. J Neurooncol 2004;66(3):313–25.

[83] Tangjitgamol S, Levenback CF, Beller U, et al. Role of surgical resection for lung, liver, and central nervous system metastases in patients with gynecological cancer: a literature review. Int J Gynecol Cancer 2004;14(3):399–422.

[84] Nakagawa K, Tago M, Terahara A, et al. A single institutional outcome analysis of Gamma Knife radiosurgery for single or multiple brain metastases. Clin Neurol Neurosurg 2000;102(4):227–32.

[85] Bartelt S, Lutterbach J. Brain metastases in patients with cancer of unknown primary. J Neurooncol 2003;64(3):249–53.

[86] Agazzi S, Pampallona S, Pica A, et al. The origin of brain metastases in patients with an undiagnosed primary tumour. Acta Neurochir (Wien) 2004;146(2):153–7.

[87] Nguyen LN, Maor MH, Oswald MJ. Brain metastases as the only manifestation of an undetected primary tumor. Cancer 1998;83(10):2181–4.

[88] Maesawa S, Kondziolka D, Thompson TP, et al. Brain metastases in patients with no known primary tumor. Cancer 2000;89(5):1095–101.

ELSEVIER
SAUNDERS

SURGICAL
CLINICS OF
NORTH AMERICA

Surg Clin N Am 85 (2005) 347–357

Palliative Care and Orthopedics: What is on the Horizon?

Dennis O. Sagini, MD[a], Albert J. Aboulafia, MD, FACS[b,c,*]

[a]Howard University Hospital, 2041 Georgia Avenue NW, Washington DC 20060, USA
[b]Alvin & Lois Lapidus Cancer Institute, Sinai Hospital of Baltimore,
2401 West Belvedere Avenue, Baltimore, MD 21215, USA
[c]Department of Orthopaedics, University of Maryland Medical School, Baltimore, MD, USA

The patient-centered model of palliative care relies on effective and empathetic communication with the goal of improving the quality of life for individuals who have terminal illness [1]. To achieve this goal, the orthopedic surgeon must be aware of the various treatment options that are available to patients who have metastatic bone disease when treating physical needs as well as increased emotional distress [2]. This includes operative and nonoperative treatment strategies; however, even if the physician is aware of the most sophisticated treatment strategies and has considerable expertise in these techniques, this qualifies him/her only as a competent technician. Providing palliative care requires more than technical expertise and knowledge.

The orthopedic surgeon's primary role in treating patients who have skeletal metastases is to improve the patient's quality of life. How one determines quality of life can be difficult. The surgeon's measure of the success of a given treatment and its effect on quality of life may differ dramatically from the patient's measure. As a general rule, the surgeon's role should be one of being a supportive facilitator by informing patients of currently available treatments, risks, and benefits. Considerations for what can and should be done for a given patient should be based primarily on the wishes of the patient and family. At times, the physician's preferred treatment plan may conflict with the patient's wishes. Ultimately, the surgeon must understand the goals of treatment from the patient's perspective and act as

---

* Corresponding author. Alvin & Lois Lapidus Cancer Institute, Emory Sinai Hospital of Baltimore, 2401 West Belvedere Avenue, Baltimore, MD 21215.
E-mail address: aaboulaf@lifebridgehealth.org (A.J. Aboulafia).

the patient's agent. The patient's right to refuse treatment should be honored. The physician should provide information to the patient and his/her family but respect the fact that the final decision regarding treatment remains with the patient. This notion seems so obvious that it might not be worthy of mention to some; however, all too often, the decision to proceed with a given treatment plan is decided before consultation with the patient and without an understanding of what and who determines measures of quality of life improvement. Patients may be informed of the recommended treatment based on the physician's best intentions to improve the patient's quality of life without understanding the patient's wishes [3,4]. It is imperative to discuss thoroughly the realistic expectations and outcomes of treatment with patients so that they can decide what risks they are willing to accept and what measures of success are meaningful to them.

The decision-making process, when treating patients who have incurable illness and associated metastatic bone disease, is an evolving area in orthopedic practice. This is true with respect to technical advances and philosophical approaches. Not long ago the classic teaching was to not operate on patients who had metastatic bone lesions unless there was an expectation that their survival was at least 3 months. This reflects an approach that is contradictory to the current recommendations of palliative care. For one, it implies that a decision regarding treatment can be made without recognizing the patient's desires. Secondly, even patients who have less than 3 months to live can benefit greatly from a treatment that allows them to be free of the side effects of narcotics and able to carry out activities that they want before their death. The notion of having patients remain bed-ridden and in pain for the terminal 3 months of their life (or even less) is no longer the only option [5–7]. The arbitrary designation of expected survival of a minimum of 3 months as a prerequisite to surgical intervention has no place in the current philosophy regarding palliative care. The objectives of treatment are, above all, to honor the patient's dignity as well as to relieve the suffering of the patient [4,8]. Crucial to maintaining a sense of dignity is maintaining the patient's ability to be autonomous in decision making and as independent as possible with daily activities. Because many pathologic bone conditions are painful, debilitating, and have poor healing potential, patients may suffer physical and psychologic symptoms that significantly diminish their quality of life [3].

General considerations

Optimal care of patients who have metastatic bone disease requires establishing clearly defined goals of treatment by the physician and the patient. Some of the goals of treatment can be measured objectively and have been used as a measure of quality of life. Other goals, such as the patient's desire to go to a movie, visit out of town family, attend a wedding, or simply attend to legal and financial matters, are more difficult to measure but may be just as important to improve the patient's quality of life as more objective measures. Goals of treatment that can be measured objectively include avoiding impending fracture, restoring function when fracture occurs, controlling local disease, and alleviating pain. This allows patients increased independence and minimizes complications of the primary disease process and it is hoped that it improves quality of life. In many cases, orthopedic surgeons are called upon to intervene surgically to realize these goals; however, patients who have metastatic disease are more prone to surgical complications than patients who do not have metastatic disease. Successful treatment requires different skills than the treatment of patients who have nonpathologic fractures. Complications of treatment or failure to achieve the goals of treatment may result from failure to recognize that a fracture is the result of a metastatic process or from treating pathologic fractures in a similar fashion as traumatic fractures.

Recently, advances in surgical techniques and implants and new medical options have improved the management of patients who have metastatic bone disease. Additionally, a better understanding of fracture risk allows more timely and accurate treatment of impending pathologic fractures, thereby preventing pathologic fractures and unnecessary prophylactic surgery. Improved operative treatments, implants and reconstruction options, and a better understanding of tumor biology and the patient who has a tumor have contributed to improved palliative care. Emerging technologies include less invasive treatment options, such as radiofrequency thermal ablation (RFA), percutaneous cementation, and the use of Cyber-Knife (Accuray, Sunnyvale, California) radiation; these may prove to be beneficial in providing palliative care for patients with skeletal metastases.

Treatment of impending pathologic fractures

Various treatment options exist for patients who have impending pathologic fractures. These include operative and nonoperative modalities. Selecting the most appropriate treatment for a given patient requires an understanding of the goals of treatment, tumor biology, and the potential advantages and limitations of the different treatment options. Pathologic fractures result from a weakening of the structural integrity of bone as a result of the effects of the tumor and usually occur during normal activity or minor trauma. Preventing pathologic fractures—rather than treating them after they occur—was shown to improve survival time and the patient's quality of life as measured by functional outcomes [5,9–11]. Estimation of fracture risk can be difficult, however. Previous guidelines that were used to assess fracture risk did not include factors, such as the patient's symptoms or histology. More recently, Mirels scoring system has been introduced which includes four criteria to assess fracture risk. The criteria include: pain (mild, moderate, severe), site (nonweight bearing, weight bearing, peritrochanteric), size (compared with bone diameter in one third increments), and type of lesion (lytic, mixed, blastic). A score of 1, 2, or 3, based on the severity of the radiographic and clinical data, is assigned to each of the four categories and the sum is calculated. The data suggest that patients who have a sum score of 8 and greater exhibit an increased risk of subsequent pathologic fracture and the need for prophylactic stabilization before radiation, whereas scores of 7 and less can be treated initially with nonoperative methods (eg, radiation) [12].

Nonoperative treatment options include the use of bisphosphonates [13]. Originally approved by the U.S. Food and Drug Administration (FDA) to reduce the incidence of skeletal complications in patients who had multiple myeloma and metastatic breast cancer, bisphosphonates may prove to be beneficial for patients who have a variety of skeletal metastases. Aridia and Zometa are bisphosphonates that are available to reduce skeletal complications, including pathologic fracture and hypercalcemia. Recent studies showed a decreased incidence of skeletally-related events for patients who had metastatic breast cancer or multiple myeloma [14]. Nonoperative treatment options are used most commonly to prevent pathologic fracture. If fracture has occurred, nonoperative treatment for long bones rarely is indicated. In cases in which fracture has occurred, the poor potential for these pathologic fractures to heal without surgery usually favors operative treatment. Prolonged immobilization in this setting usually results in impaired function and persistent pain, and adversely affects quality of life (Fig. 1).

Nonoperative palliative treatment of pathologic bone disease also includes the use of radiation therapy. The most common form is external beam radiation [15]. Recently, stereotactic radiation with the CyberKnife was applied to patients who had metastatic bone lesions. The CyberKnife offers the potential of delivering extremely high doses of radiation to a much-focused area, thus minimizing excess radiation to surrounding tissue and structures. Additionally, compared with conventional radiation therapy, the CyberKnife requires fewer treatments and usually can be completed within 5 days (versus 2–5 weeks for conventional treatments). There is no literature on the long-term outcomes that compare the survival, local tumor control, and pain relief of patients who were treated using the CyberKnife with conventional external beam radiation.

Principles of operative treatment

Pathologic fractures are biologically different from fractures that result from trauma. As a result, applying the same principles to fracture care in metastatic disease as in trauma results in a higher incidence of complications. Common complications in the operative treatment of pathologic fracture include delayed healing and nonunion. The treatment of non-pathologic fractures relies on the concept of initial stabilization to provide mechanical support and alignment until the fracture heals. In pathologic

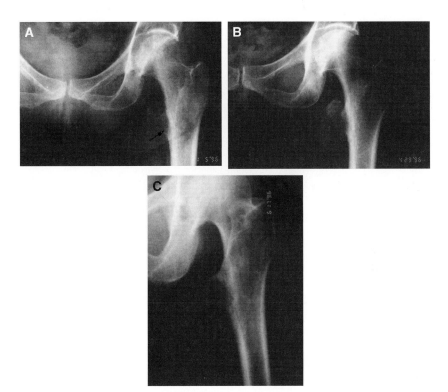

Fig. 1. This 56-year-old woman had breast cancer 18 years earlier. She developed acute pain in the left hip. After unsuccessful prolonged nonoperative treatment due to failure to diagnose and then failure to understand the poor potential for pathologic fractures to heal, she was referred for operative treatment. (*A*) Radiographs of the left hip reveal an avulsion fracture of the lesser trochanter. The radiograph is pathomnemonic for a pathologic fracture. Despite the history of breast cancer, it was not recognized as being pathologic and the patient was prescribed crutches and oral narcotics (arrow indicates site of fracture). (*B*) Radiograph taken more than 3 months later shows no evidence of healing. Patient was now unable to walk and was confined to a wheel chair. (*C*) Five and one half months after her initial presentation, the suspected diagnosis of metastatic breast cancer was made and radiation was recommended. (*D*) After completing radiation, the patient was still wheelchair bound, was on high dosages of narcotics, and was unable to get from her bed to a chair without assistance. She required an ambulance to get to the doctor's office for this radiograph, which revealed progressive disease. No palliative treatments were discussed with the patient. (*E*) Nearly 15 months later the patient was referred to an orthopedic surgeon for operative treatment. After discussing treatment options, she underwent hip replacement surgery and was weaned completely from narcotics and was an independent ambulator.

fractures, however, because of the biology of the tumor and other factors, the bone never heals and the hardware ultimately fails. Delay or failure of the bone to heal increases the stress that implants must bear; after numerous cycles, this results in microfracture and failure [16]. Therefore, the selection of the method of fixation for pathologic fractures is different than for

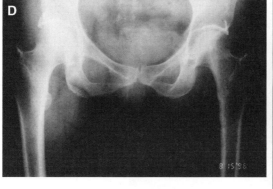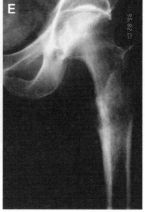

Fig. 1 (*continued*)

nonpathologic fractures. Specifically, the treatment goal for traumatic fracture is to stabilize and preserve the milieu to allow the fracture to heal. In many cases, the construct is designed to allow the gradual return of function over several weeks until the bone heals. In contrast, the treatment goal of pathologic fractures is to allow immediate return of function with a construct that does not rely on fracture healing (Fig. 2).

Highest failure rates after surgical stabilization are observed in patients who have metastatic renal cell carcinoma (24%) or distal femoral lesions (20%). Failure rates for fractures that are treated with standard osteosynthesis techniques (plates and screws) are associated with failure rates of approximately 15%. Endoprostheses (use of an implant that replaces the bone) are associated with much lower failure rates of approximately 2% to 5%. Therefore, surgeons must select a surgical procedure that achieves the goals of immediate stability and pain relief, is durable enough to last the patient's lifetime, and does not rely on fracture healing.

General principles that are unique to oncologic fracture care include the use of adjuvants postoperatively (eg, radiation, chemotherapy) to minimize the chance of local tumor progression (Fig. 3). Additionally, fixation techniques that "protect" the entire length of the involved bone should be selected. Often, a proximal lesion is stabilized only to have the patient develop a fracture distal to the previous fracture (Fig. 4). In selected cases, a radical resection with wide excision and reconstruction using a modular prosthesis may be more appropriate than attempting to stabilize a fracture. Whether due to poor bone quality or local recurrence, many periprosthetic fractures may be avoided if a long-stem prosthesis is selected. This concept is especially important in patients who have long life expectancies and those who have a high probability of additional metastasis (eg, breast and renal cancers).

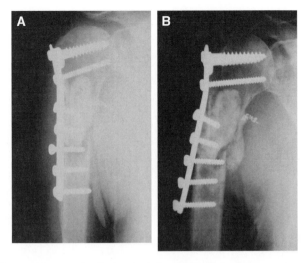

Fig. 2. A 52-year-old man who had metastatic renal cell carcinoma underwent operative treatment for a pathologic humerus fracture. (*A*) Postoperative radiograph show internal fixation hardware supplemented with polymethylmethacrylate (PMMA). (*B*) Despite the use of PMMA, the construct fails because the fracture never heals. The coils indicate preoperative embolization.

Future directions in palliative care

Patients who have metastatic disease who are poor surgical candidates or who have multiple comorbidities may not be able to survive lengthy operative procedures. These patients generally have hemodynamic and metabolic considerations and cannot tolerate prolonged anesthesia time, excessive blood loss, or a lengthy hospital stay. In these cases, patients may benefit from a minimally invasive procedure, such as cementoplasty, RFA, or a combination of cementoplasty and RFA.

Cementoplasty has been used in the past for stabilization of osteoporotic compression fractures in the spine; it is approved by the FDA for this indication. In the spine, opacified bone cement is injected slowly into an osseous void percutaneously under continuous fluoroscopic guidance. The goals of the procedure are to increase the stability of the osteoporotic bone, relieve pain, and prevent progressive deformity. Studies to investigate the application of this technique to patients who have osseous voids that were created by metastatic disease are underway [11,16]. This may prove to be especially useful for patients who have pelvic or spinal lesions [17]. Its application for lesions in long bones has not been studied.

RFA has been used to treat a variety of extraskeletal malignant conditions, including hepatic tumors (primary and metastatic), cardiac arrhythmias, renal cell carcinomas, recurrent rectal carcinoma, and unresectable pulmonary tumors (primary and metastatic). In the skeleton, RFA was highly effective for the treatment of osteoid osteomas, a benign bone tumor

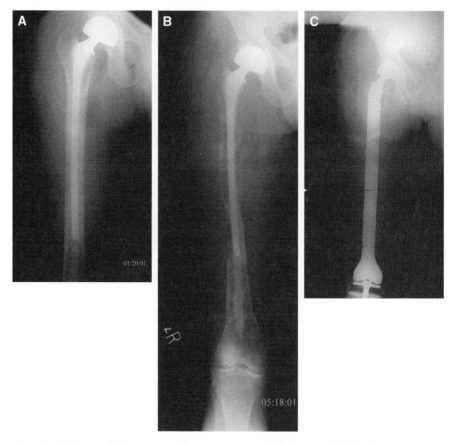

Fig. 3. A 52-year-old intravenous drug user was treated for a pathologic fracture of the proximal femur resulting from metastatic lung cancer but refused postoperative radiation and chemotherapy. (*A*) Initial postoperative radiograph shows hip replacement with a long-stem prosthesis. (*B*) Four months later the patient returned with severe pain and inability to walk. Radiographs demonstrated massive osteolysis and tumor progression. (*C*) A total femoral replacement was performed for palliation. The patient died of disease 2 months later but was pain free and was an independent ambulator.

that most commonly affects children or young adults. Given the successful results of treatment of malignant tumors in extraskeletal locations and the application for treatment of benign bone lesions, RFA was used recently to treat skeletal metastases. RFA may be combined with cementoplasty in an effort to control local disease and achieve immediate stability and pain relief (Fig. 5). The technique involves using an 18-gauge radionics RF probe with a 5-mm active tip that is inserted through an Ackerman needle under fluoroscopic or CT guidance. There are limited data available regarding the use of RFA and cementoplasty in palliating patients who have bone metastases. A summary of three series of patients who were treated

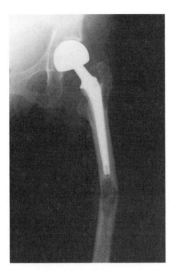

Fig. 4. A 66-year-old woman who had breast cancer was treated for a pathologic femoral neck fracture using "standard" operative methods for nonpathologic fracture. Radiograph 4 months later demonstrates a fracture at the tip of the prosthesis. Failure to protect the entire bone resulted in subsequent fracture and need for revision surgery.

with cementoplasty and consisted of 42 acetabular, 4 sacral, and 2 iliac lesions demonstrated 83% pain relief and local recurrence in 13% of patients.

Cementoplasty and RFA are not in wide clinical use. Their application, indications, risks, benefits, and long-term results remain to be defined [17].

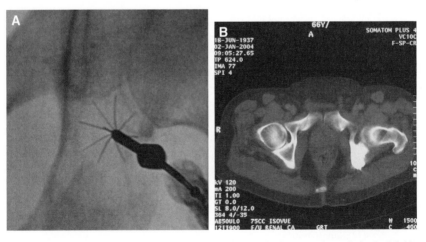

Fig. 5. A 66-year-old man who had metastatic renal cancer had progressive pain in the left hip. (A) RFA was performed for a lesion that involved the inferior pubic ramus and inferior posterior acetabulum. The probe fills the majority of the lesion. (B) Following RFA, PMMA was introduced into the lesion. Complete filling of the lesion is demonstrated on CT scan.

Other methods that are under investigation include adding chemotherapeutic agents (eg, methotrexate) to polymethylmethacrylate, the bone cement that is used in orthopedic surgery.

Summary

Patient-centered palliative care involves effective and empathetic communication between the physician and patient, with the ultimate goal of providing improved quality of life for individuals who have terminal illnesses. Although several nonoperative and operative treatment options are available to improve the patient's quality of life, providing palliative care requires more than technical expertise and knowledge. Orthopedic surgeons need to be supportive facilitators who inform patients of the available treatments, risks, and benefits and incorporate these treatments into the wishes of patients and their families. Realistic expectations and outcomes of treatment need to be discussed with patients so that they can decide what risks they are willing to accept and what measures of success are meaningful to them. Advances in medical treatments and surgical techniques and principles are available to patients who have metastatic bone disease that were not available less than a decade ago. Although many orthopedic surgeons are involved in the care of patients who have metastatic disease, at times, expertise from an orthopedic oncologist may be required to optimize palliative care.

References

[1] Dunn GP, Milch RA. Is this a bad day, or one of the last days? How to recognize and respond to approaching demise. J Am Coll Surg 2002;195(6):879–87.
[2] Aaronson NK, Ahmedzai S, Bergman B. The European Organization for Research and Treatment of Cancer QLQ-C30: a quality-of-life instrument for use in international clinical trials in oncology. J Natl Cancer Inst 1993;85(5):365–76.
[3] Dunn GP. Patient assessment in palliative care: how to see the "big picture" and what to do when "there is no more we can do." J Am Coll Surg 2001;193(5):565–73.
[4] Dunn GP, Milch RA. Introduction and historical background of palliative care: where does the surgeon fit in? J Am Coll Surg 2001;193(3):325–8.
[5] Broos PL, Rommens PM, Vanlangenaker MJ. Pathological fractures of the femur: improvement of quality of life after surgical treatment. Arch Orthop Trauma Surg 1992; 111(2):73–7.
[6] Harrington KD. Orthopedic surgical management of skeletal complications of malignancy. Cancer 1997;80(8)(Suppl):1614–27.
[7] Healey JH, Brown HK. Complications of bone metastases: surgical management. Cancer 2000;88(12)(Suppl):2940–51.
[8] Dunn GP, Milch RA, Mosenthal AC, et al. Palliative care by the surgeon: how to do it. J Am Coll Surg 2002;194:509–37.
[9] Lee SH, Kim HS, Kim SR, et al. Functional outcome following surgical treatment of metastatic tumors involving the femur. Orthopedics 2000;23(10):1075–9.

[10] Hardman PD, Robb JE, Kerr GR, et al. The value of internal fixation and radiotherapy in the management of upper and lower limb bone metastases. Clin Oncol (R Coll Radiol) 1992; 4(4):244–8.

[11] Van Geffen E, Wobbes T, Veth RP, et al. Operative management of impending pathological fractures: a critical analysis of therapy. J Surg Oncol 1997;64(3):190–4.

[12] Mirels H. Metastatic disease in long bones. A proposed system for diagnosing impending pathologic fractures. Clin Orthop 1989;249:256–64.

[13] Mercadante S. Malignant bone pain: pathophysiology and treatment. Pain 1997;69(1–2): 1–18.

[14] Perry CM, Figgitt DP. Zoledronic acid: a review of its use in patients with advanced cancer. Drugs 2004;(11):1197–211.

[15] Gaze MN, Kelly CG, Kerr GR, et al. Pain relief and quality of life following radiotherapy for bone metastases: a randomized trial of two fractionation schedules. Radiother Oncol 1997; 45(2):109–16.

[16] Dijstra S, Wiggers T, van Geel BN, et al. Impending and actual pathological fractures in patients with bone metastases of the long bones. A retrospective study of 233 surgically treated fractures. Eur J Surg 1994;160(10):535–42.

[17] Jacofsky DJ, Papagelopoulos PJ, Sim FH. Advances and challenges in the surgical treatment of metastatic bone disease. Clin Orthop 2003;415(Suppl):S14–8.

SURGICAL
CLINICS OF
NORTH AMERICA

Surg Clin N Am 85 (2005) 359–371

Palliative Therapy for Pancreatic/Biliary Cancer

Michael G. House, MD[a], Michael A. Choti, MD[b],*

[a]Department of Surgery, The Johns Hopkins University School of Medicine,
600 North Wolfe Street, Baltimore, MD 21287, USA
[b]Division of Surgical Oncology, The Johns Hopkins University School of Medicine,
600 North Wolfe Street, Halsted 614, Baltimore, MD 21287, USA

Pancreatic cancer, with an annual incidence of approximately 28,000 cases, is the fourth leading cause of cancer-related mortality in men and women in the United States. Bile duct cancer is much less common, affecting only 2500 individuals each year [1]. Despite advances in surgical treatment and medical and radiation therapy, the overall prognosis for these malignancies remains quite poor. Unfortunately, at the time of initial diagnosis, only 50% of patients with pancreatic cancer are free of distant metastases, and only 20% of these patients have localized disease amenable to curative resection [2,3]. Likewise, the resectability rate for extrahepatic cholangiocarcinoma remains low, ranging between 40% and 60% [4]. Even though most patients with pancreatic or bile duct cancer are not candidates for curative surgical resection because of early metastatic spread or extensive local tumor involvement, palliation of obstructive symptoms and pain remains a core component in the management of these diseases. Depending on performance status and medical comorbidities, survival for patients with metastatic disease is on the order of 3 to 6 months, whereas patients with nonmetastatic, locally advanced cancer experience a median survival on the order of 6 to 12 months [5–7]. Regardless of the dismal survival in most cases, every attempt, whether nonoperative or operative, should be made to improve the quality of life for patients with unresectable cancer of the pancreas or bile duct.

Palliative treatment for unresectable periampullary cancer, including cancers of the pancreatic head, distal common bile duct, duodenum, and ampulla, is directed at three major symptoms: (1) obstructive jaundice, (2)

[This article was originally published in *Clinics in Sports Medicine* 7:1, January 1988.]
* Corresponding author.
E-mail address: mchoti@jhmi.edu (M.A. Choti).

duodenal obstruction, and (3) cancer-related pain. For hilar cholangiocarcinoma, palliation of biliary obstruction to prevent secondary hepatic failure is a primary management goal, whereas, cholangiocarcinoma of the intrahepatic bile ducts typically is managed as a liver mass and is not discussed further in this article. In the past, surgical treatment has traditionally served as the principal modality for palliating the symptoms associated with locally advanced periampullary cancer; however, improved nonoperative strategies, including endoluminal biliary and duodenal stents and minimally invasive celiac plexus blockade, have gained popularity in the management of patients with definitively unresectable disease, particularly those with limited performance status, significant cardiopulmonary disease, or coexistent liver cirrhosis [8–14]. Even though assessment of tumor unresectability has been enhanced by recent advances in CT and MRI as well as by the selective use of percutaneous transhepatic cholangiography (PTC) and diagnostic laparoscopy, open surgical exploration continues to serve as the standard for determining tumor resectability. For patients undergoing open exploration for potentially resectable pancreatic or bile duct cancer, surgical palliation is often indicated when nonmetastatic, unresectable disease is found intraoperatively [5,6,10]. In most cases, the pattern of symptoms at the time of diagnosis in the context of the patient's medical condition and projected survival influence the decision to perform an operative versus a nonoperative palliative procedure (Fig. 1).

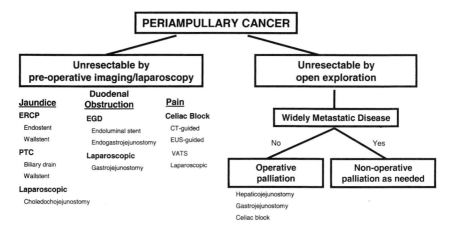

Fig. 1. The use of various modalities for palliating periampullary cancer depends on the location of the unresectable disease. Nonoperative procedures are performed as symptoms develop in patients with unresectable disease determined by noninvasive means. For patients with unresectable disease at the time of laparotomy, operative palliation for the three major cancer-related symptoms should be performed except in patients with limited projected survival (ie, those with widely metastatic disease).

Obstructive jaundice

Two thirds of cholangiocarcinomas are perihilar and another 25% arise from the distal common bile duct. Thus, the most common symptom associated with cholangiocarcinoma is painless jaundice [15]. Approximately three quarters of exocrine neoplasms of the pancreas arise in the head of the pancreas. Consequently, 65% to 75% of patients with pancreatic adenocarcinoma seek medical attention for symptoms related to jaundice secondary to mechanical obstruction of the intrapancreatic portion of the distal common bile duct [5]. Obstructive jaundice can also be accompanied by refractory pruritus, anorexia, malabsorptive diarrhea, and progressive malnutrition, all of which can lead to generalized wasting. If left untreated, biliary obstruction can result in cholangitis or metabolic and synthetic liver dysfunction that can precipitate early death. For these reasons, decompression of biliary obstruction leads to a dramatic improvement in the overall medical condition that contributes to a prolongation of comfortable survival [16].

Endoscopic and percutaneous palliation

For jaundiced patients with definitively unresectable pancreatic or bile duct cancer found on preoperative evaluation, nonoperative palliative therapy is generally indicated. Since its clinical inception in 1980, the use of endoscopically placed biliary endoprostheses has continued to evolve and now serves as the predominant modality for palliating obstructive jaundice [17]. In most cases, endoscopic palliation is preferable to percutaneous palliation for malignant biliary obstruction because it allows definitive internal drainage with one procedure. With experience and standardized equipment, biliary drainage can be accomplished successfully with a 10-F endoprosthesis in more than 90% of patients during endoscopic retrograde cholangiopancreatography (ERCP) [18,19]. Endoscopic attempts at biliary drainage fail in fewer than 10% of patients with periampullary tumors, including distal cholangiocarcinoma and pancreatic cancer. In these cases, technical failures usually result from tumor infiltration into the duodenal wall that prevents access to the ampulla [18]. In the event that endoscopic management is unsuccessful or not possible, PTC should be performed to accomplish external biliary drainage (Fig. 2).

For more proximal hilar biliary cancers (Bismuth type II, III, and IV cholangiocarcinoma) the success rate of endoscopic stent decompression is only approximately 50% and largely reflects technical experience [20]. Despite technical difficulty, insertion of a plastic biliary endoprosthesis is the most common method used by experienced endoscopists to palliate hilar obstruction. With regards to the relative merits of unilateral versus bilateral stenting for advanced hilar cholangiocarcinoma, recent prospective studies

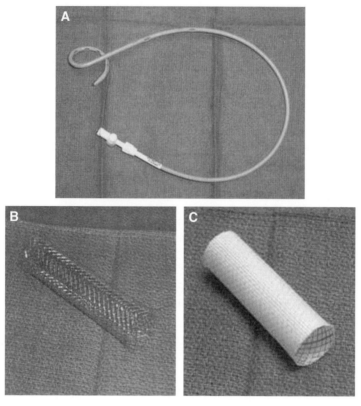

Fig. 2. Percutaneous biliary drainage devices. (*A*) Silastic biliary drainage catheter (Flexima), (*B*) bare metallic biliary stent, (*C*) metallic bilary endostent covered with PTFE.

have failed to demonstrate any improvements in outcomes or complications with the routine use of bilateral stents for unresectable hilar tumors [20]. Therefore, the decision to place one or more biliary stents is determined by the extent of opacification of the biliary tree at the time of cholangiography [20–22].

Silastic endoprostheses and particularly percutaneous biliary catheters require repeat manipulations to maintain patency and prevent cholangitis. Therefore, primary or delayed placement of a self-expanding metallic stent has become preferable for unresectable patients in whom palliative interventions alone are appropriate (Fig. 2). Although metallic stents afford significantly better long-term patency compared with endoprostheses (9 months versus 4 months), occlusions can occur with tumor ingrowth [23]. For this reason, novel biliary stents, incorporating an impermeable sheath or cytotoxic compounds, recently have been developed to avoid complications of reocclusion [24]. Furthermore, most clinicians are uncomfortable placing metallic biliary stents during the initial endoscopic or percutaneous procedure, particularly if a definitive opinion regarding resectability has not been rendered [25]. In most circumstances, metallic stents are deployed at the time of a remanipulation of an existing biliary drainage catheter. Another advantage of metal over plastic stents for the management of hilar tumors is the open mesh design, which has the potential for permitting continued patency of the contralateral ducts, which would otherwise be occluded by the closed-wall stent.

Surgical palliation

Surgical palliation of obstructive jaundice is indicated for patients with biliary or pancreatic cancer that is determined to be unresectable only at the time of exploratory laparotomy or laparoscopy or for patients in relatively good medical condition with expected survival beyond 3 to 6 months, particularly when nonoperative palliation is not successful. In most cases, patients with unresectable periampullary cancer or distal cholangiocarcinoma should undergo surgical biliary bypass. Alternatively, one may consider not performing a biliary bypass at the time of surgical exploration, relying on endoscopic or percutaneous decompression. This question remains controversial among surgeons, particularly when successful biliary decompression was not accomplished preoperatively.

The optimal surgical biliary bypass is the choledochojejunostomy. Cholecystojejunostomy is associated with a lower success rate for palliating jaundice than bypass to the common duct and should generally be avoided if at all possible [10,26,27]. In most cases, choledochojejunostomy can be accomplished with either a simple jejunal loop or a Roux-en-Y limb (Fig. 3). Although a loop anastomosis requires slightly less operative time, the use of a defunctionalized Roux-en-Y jejunal limb is associated with less anastomotic tension and facilitates the management of potential biliary leaks. Also, the incidence of postoperative cholangitis seems to be reduced with Roux limb drainage.

Unlike periampullary cancer, surgical palliation for obstructive jaundice from hilar cholangiocarcinoma has a limited role. Although tumor debulking with hepaticojejunostomy offers a reliable way to palliate jaundice, this surgical approach should be reserved for tumors that are determined to be unresectable after extensive dissection of the hilar structures, including transection of one or more bile ducts [4]. Alternatively, a bilioenteric anastomosis to segment III or right sectorial ducts for left or right sided biliary obstruction, respectively, can also be performed to accomplish biliary decompression. Unlike right-side decompression, bypass to segment III is easier to perform and is the favored approach in most cases. When performing this procedure, the dilated duct is identified within the hepatic parenchyma. The segment III duct can be identified adjacent to the segmental portal vein branch, just to the left of the falciform ligament. The duct is incised over a distance of about 1 cm and

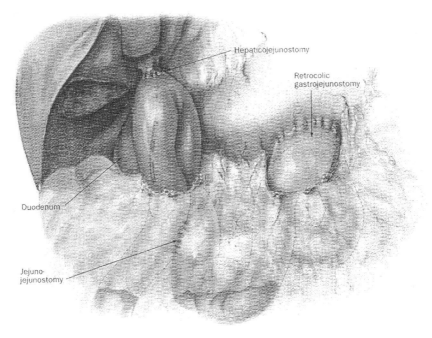

Fig. 3. Operative palliation for obstructive jaundice and duodenal obstruction. Here, the biliary obstruction is bypassed with a retrocolic loop (end-to-side) hepaticojejunostomy in continuity with a loop gastrojejunostomy. A side-to-side jejuno-jejunostomy is added to limit biliary reflux into the stomach. As an alternative, the hepaticojejunostomy can be performed with a Roux-en-Y limb (not shown) procedure.

anastomosed side-to-side to a Roux-en-Y loop of jejunum. This procedure, while effective at biliary decompression, is associated with increased morbidity compared with nonsurgical palliation and is not commonly indicated.

Median survival after surgical palliation of obstructive jaundice secondary to pancreatic adenocarcinoma is approximately 5 to 6 months and, in general, does not depend on the type of procedure performed [28–31]. Interestingly, the addition of surgical biliary decompression, alone, to exploratory laparotomy for unresectable pancreatic cancer has been shown to improve survival by as much as 2 months. Compared with nonoperative techniques, which carry a lower short-term morbidity, mortality, hospital stay, and cost, the major advantage of surgical biliary bypass is the lower incidence of late complications, namely recurrent jaundice and cholangitis (Table 1) [5,6,16]. Although the increased use of expandable metallic stents has lowered the incidence of recurrent jaundice, late complications develop in approximately 25% of patients undergoing various forms of nonoperative palliation [32–36]. In comparison, fewer than 10% of patients undergoing operative biliary drainage develop late complications [5–7].

Table 1
Prospective comparison between endoscopic stenting and surgical bypass in patients with malignant biliary obstruction

	Surgery	Stenting	P value
Total patients	101	100	
Therapeutic success	92%	92%	NS
Complications			
Major	29%	11%	0.02
Minor	29%	18%	NS
Mortality			
Procedure-related	14%	3%	0.06
30-day	15%	8%	NS
Median hospital stay (d)	26	19	NS
Median overall survival (wks)	26	21	NS

From Smith AC, Dowsett JF, Russell RC, Hatfield AR, Cotton PB. Randomised trial of endoscopic stenting versus surgical bypass in malignant low bile duct obstruction. Lancet 1994; 344:1655–60; with permission.

Duodenal obstruction

As many as 30% to 50% of patients with periampullary cancer, especially pancreatic head cancer, have nausea and vomiting at the time of their initial diagnosis even though demonstrable radiographic evidence of duodenal obstruction is documented in only a small fraction of these patients [37]. Moreover, with disease progression within the periampullary region, up to one third of patients eventually develop true mechanical obstruction along the duodenal C-loop [37]. In large retrospective studies of patients who did not undergo prophylactic gastrojejunostomy as part of a surgical procedure, between 10% and 25% of them developed obstructive symptoms requiring subsequent operative gastrojejunostomy, and an additional 20% eventually died with duodenal obstruction [37,38].

Surgical palliation

When pancreatic cancer is determined to be unresectable at the time of exploratory laparotomy or laparoscopy, prophylactic gastrojejunostomy should be performed in most cases, unless a life expectancy of less than 3 to 6 months is anticipated based on intraoperative findings [37]. Although routine gastrojejunostomy adds to operative time, it does not contribute to postoperative morbidity or mortality or length of hospital stay. In the past, most surgeons advocated an antecolic gastrojejunostomy because of concerns of placing the anastomosis in proximity to the tumor bed; however, there is now strong evidence that a retrocolic, isoperistaltic gastrojejunostomy is associated with a lower incidence of postoperative delayed gastric emptying and even late occurring gastric outlet obstruction [36]. The anastomosis should be fashioned at the most dependent aspect of the greater curvature of the stomach with a loop of jejunum approximately

30 cm from the ligament of Treitz. In most cases, Roux-en-Y reconstruction is not necessary. Vagotomy is generally avoided during palliative gastro-jejunostomy to prevent delayed gastric emptying (Fig. 3). Thus, all patients should be maintained long-term on either histamine H_2-blockers or proton pump inhibitors to prevent marginal ulceration at the anastomosis.

Endoscopic palliation

Although palliation of duodenal or gastric outlet obstruction tradition-ally has been managed surgically, there has been growing interest in endoluminal approaches to relieving obstruction. In the past, endoscopic options included tube gastrostomy with jejunal extension for nutritional access; however, the development of self-expanding enteral stents with a luminal diameter between 2 and 3 cm provides a reliable, nonsurgical method for palliating duodenal obstruction in patients who do not require surgical exploration to determine resectability. Despite early success with enteral stents in small series, complications can arise. These include mucosal ulceration, duodenal perforation, stent migration, and tumor ingrowth leading to recurrent obstruction [38]. Patients with reasonable life expec-tancy who fail endoscopic attempts at palliation or develop complications related to endoluminal stenting may require surgical gastrojejunostomy [38].

Cancer-related pain

Pain related to pancreatic cancer is perhaps the most debilitating symptom associated with this disease and can quickly lead to the deterioration of the patient's quality of life and performance status. For this reason, palliative care must concentrate on adequate pain control. Although only 30% to 40% of patients with pancreatic cancer report moderate to severe pain at the time of diagnosis, more than 80% of patients with advanced cancer experience severe pain before death [39,40]. The two primary methods for treating pancreatic cancer-related pain involve systemic analgesics and regional neurolysis. Involved nerves in the region of the celiac plexus harbor sympathetic afferent nerve fibers transmitting nociceptive information from the pancreas. In the past, a celiac plexus block was reserved for patients who failed opioid analgesics. Early implementation of a celiac plexus nerve block before the onset of incapacitating pain, however, has been shown to be more effective in maintaining overall quality of life [39]. There are generally four techniques used to achieve a disruption of the splanchnic nerves by celiac block: (1) intraoperative chemical splanchnicectomy, (2) percutaneous celiac plexus block, (3) endoscopically guided celiac plexus block, and (4) thoracoscopic splanchnicectomy [39–41]. Since its introduction in 1978, chemical splanchni-cectomy has been used to palliate pain in patients found to be unresectable at the time of exploratory laparotomy. Typically, this procedure is performed concomitantly with palliative biliary and gastrointestinal bypass and involves the injection of 20 mL of 50% alcohol on each side of the aorta at the level of the celiac axis. Chemical splanchnicectomy can achieve acute pain relief in more than 80% of patients and can prevent the subsequent onset of pain for up to 6 months postoperatively [39]. Furthermore, patients with severe preoperative pain who later undergo a palliative chemical splanchnicectomy experience a significant improvement in overall survival (Fig. 4). For these reasons, chemical splanchnicectomy should be considered in all patients with preoperative pain who are determined to be unresectable at the time of exploratory laparotomy and at least considered even in those who are anticipated to have pain problems postoperatively.

Unresectable patients who do not undergo laparotomy usually can achieve adequate analgesia with appropriate doses of both long- and short-acting opioid compounds. In some patients, pain can become intractable despite escalating doses of pharmacologic agents and can begin to interfere with activities of daily living. One adjunct to opioid medications is percutaneous celiac plexus block under CT or fluoroscopic guidance. Again, ethanol is most often used as the neurolytic agent and can interrupt nerve transmission for up to 6 months. Immediately after this procedure, 75% to 85% of patients report excellent pain control that is maintained to the end of life [40]. In some patients with bulky periaortic lymphadenopathy or disease encasing the celiac trunk, a percutaneous celiac plexus block may not be possible via the standard posterior approach. In these circumstances, one should consider either endoscopic ultrasound-guided celiac plexus neurolysis or thoracoscopic neurotomy of the splanchnic nerve branches arising from the sympathetic trunk at vertebral levels T5 through T12.

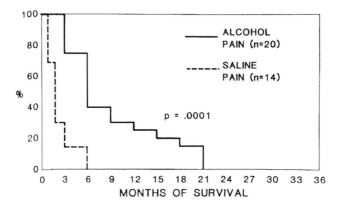

Fig. 4. Kaplan-Meier survival analysis for patients with preoperative pain. Survival is determined from the time of hospital discharge after operative chemical splanchnicectomy. (*From* Lillemoe KD, Cameron JL, Kaufman HS, Yeo CJ, Pitt HA, Sauter PK. Chemical splanchnicectomy in patients with unresectable pancreatic cancer: a prospective randomized trial. Ann Surg 1993;217(5):447–55 [discussion: 456–7]; with permission.)

Palliative pancreaticoduodenectomy

Generally, pancreaticoduodenectomy for adenocarcinoma is reserved for patients who are candidates for potentially curative resection. As post-operative morbidity continues to improve with this procedure, there is growing interest in performing pancreaticoduodenectomy with palliative intent for patients with pancreatic and periampullary cancer that cannot be resected completely with negative surgical margins. In the presence of visceral or other distant metastatic disease, pancreatectomy should still not be considered an appropriate palliative procedure, particularly when limited survival is expected. Although the role of pancreaticoduodenectomy for palliative intent remains controversial and in most cases is not recom-mended, comparative studies by Lillemoe et al [42] have shown that patients with localized disease who undergo pancreaticoduodenectomy with evidence of gross or microscopic residual disease (R1 or R2) have improved survival compared with similar patients who receive surgical palliative bypass procedures alone (Fig. 5). Although pancreaticoduodenectomy is associated with a longer length of hospital stay and a higher incidence of postoperative complications compared with palliative bypasses, palliative resection may help to avoid long-term complications necessitating further nonoperative and operative procedures and can be considered in selected situations [42].

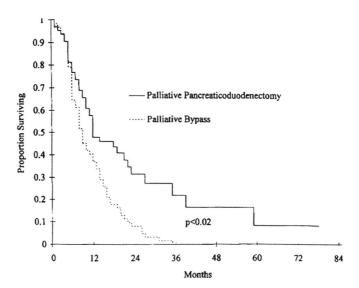

Fig. 5. Kaplan-Meier survival analysis for patients who were explored for a periampullary cancer and underwent either a palliative double bypass or a margin-positive resection. (*From* Lillemoe KD, Cameron JL, Yeo CJ, Sohn TA, Nakeeb A, Sauter PK et al. Pancreaticoduo-denectomy. Does it have a role in the palliation of pancreatic cancer? Ann Surg 1996; 223(6):718–25 [discussion: 725–8]; with permission.)

Summary

Palliative treatment for unresectable periampullary cancer is directed at three major symptoms: obstructive jaundice, duodenal obstruction, and cancer-related pain. In most cases, the pattern of symptoms at the time of diagnosis in the context of the patient's medical condition and projected survival influence the decision to perform an operative versus a nonoperative palliative procedure. Despite improvements in preoperative imaging and laparoscopic staging of patients with periampullary cancer and hilar cholangiocarcinoma, surgical exploration is the only modality that can definitively rule out resectability and the potential for curative resection in some patients with nonmetastatic cancer. Furthermore, only surgical management achieves successful palliation of obstructive symptoms and cancer-related pain as a single procedure during exploration. To take advantage of the long-term advantages afforded by surgical palliation, operative procedures must be performed with acceptable morbidity. The average postoperative length of hospital stay for patients who undergo surgical palliation is less than 15 days, even in those who develop minor complications. The average survival of patients who receive surgical palliation alone for nonmetastatic, unresectable pancreatic cancer is approximately 8 months. As with all treatment planning, palliative therapy for pancreatic and biliary cancer should be planned using a multidisciplinary approach, including input from the surgeon, gastroenterologist, radiologist, and medical and radiation oncologist. In this way, quality of life can be optimized in most patients with these diseases.

References

[1] Landis SH, Murray T, Bolden S, Wingo PA. Cancer statistics, 1999. CA Cancer J Clin 1999; 49(1):8–31.

[2] Kalser MH, Barkin J, MacIntyre JM. Pancreatic cancer: assessment of prognosis by clinical presentation. Cancer 1985;56(2):397–402.

[3] Ahrendt SA, Pitt HA. Surgical management of pancreatic cancer. Oncology (Huntingt) 2002;16(6) [discussion: 734, 736–8, 740, 743]:725–34 [discussion: 77–8].

[4] Yeo CJ, Pitt HA, Cameron JL. Cholangiocarcinoma. Surg Clinic North Am 1990;71: 1429–47.

[5] Sohn TA, Lillemoe KD, Cameron JL, Huang JJ, Pitt HA, Yeo CJ. Surgical palliation of unresectable periampullary adenocarcinoma in the 1990s. J Am Coll Surg 1999;188(6): 658–66 [discussion: 666–9].

[6] Singh SM, Longmire WP Jr, Reber HA. Surgical palliation for pancreatic cancer: the UCLA experience. Ann Surg 1990;212(2):132–9.

[7] Singh SM, Reber HA. Surgical palliation for pancreatic cancer. Surg Clin North Am 1989; 69(3):599–611.

[8] de Rooij PD, Rogatko A, Brennan MF. Evaluation of palliative surgical procedures in unresectable pancreatic cancer. Br J Surg 1991;78(9):1053–8.

[9] Di Fronzo LA, Cymerman J, Egrari S, O'Connell TX. Unresectable pancreatic carcinoma: correlating length of survival with choice of palliative bypass. Am Surg 1999; 65(10):955–8.

[10] Lillemoe KD. Palliative therapy for pancreatic cancer. Surg Oncol Clin N Am 1998;7(1): 199–216.

[11] Potts JR 3rd, Broughan TA, Hermann RE. Palliative operations for pancreatic carcinoma. Am J Surg 1990;159(1):72–7 [discussion: 77–8].

[12] Sarr MG, Cameron JL. Surgical management of unresectable carcinoma of the pancreas. Surgery 1982;91(2):123–33.

[13] Abraham S, Barkun J, Barkun A. Palliation of malignant biliary obstruction: a prospective trial examining impact on quality of life. Gastrointest Endosc 2002;56:835–41.

[14] Spanknebel K, Conlon KC. Advances in the surgical management of pancreatic cancer. Cancer J 2001;7(4):312–23.

[15] Burke EC, Jarnagin WR, Hochwald SN, Pisters PW, Fong Y, Blumgart LH. Hilar cholangiocarcinoma: patterns of spread, importance of hepatic resection for curative operation, and a presurgical clinical staging system. Ann Surg 1998;228:385–94.

[16] Brandabur JJ, Kozarek RA, Ball TJ, Hofer BO, Ryan JA Jr, Traverso LW, et al. Nonoperative versus operative treatment of obstructive jaundice in pancreatic cancer: cost and survival analysis. Am J Gastroenterol 1988;83(10):1132–9.

[17] Soehendra N, Reynders-Frederix V. Palliative bile duct drainage—a new endoscopic method of introducing a transpapillary drain. Endoscopy 1980;12(1):8–11.

[18] Arguedas MR, Heudebert GH, Stinnett AA, Wilcox CM. Biliary stents in malignant obstructive jaundice due to pancreatic carcinoma: a cost-effectiveness analysis. Am J Gastroenterol 2002;97(4):898–904.

[19] Lichtenstein DR, Carr-Locke DL. Endoscopic palliation for unresectable pancreatic carcinoma. Surg Clin North Am 1995;75(5):969–88.

[20] Chang WH, Kortan P, Haber GB. Outcome in patients with bifurcation tumors who undergo unilateral versus bilateral hepatic duct drainage. Gastrointest Endosc 1998;47:354–62.

[21] Polydorou AA, Cairns SR, Dowsett JF, Hatfield AR, Salmon PR, Cotton PB. Palliation of proximal malignant biliary obstruction by endoscopic endoprosthesis insertion. Gut 1991; 32:685–9.

[22] Deviere J, Haize M, de Toeuf J, Cremer M. Long term follow-up of patients with hilar malignant strictures treated by endoscopic internal biliary drainage. Gastrointest Endosc 1988;34:95–101.

[23] Maetani I, Ogawa S, Hoshi H, Sato M, Yoshioka H, Igarashi Y, et al. Self-expanding metal stents for palliative treatment of malignant biliary and duodenal stenoses. Endoscopy 1994; 26(8):701–4.

[24] Mezawa S, Homma H, Sato T, Doi T, Mihanishi K, Takada K, et al. A study of carboplatin-coated tube for unresectable cholangiocarcinoma. Hepatology 2000;32(5):916–23.

[25] Davids PH, Groen AK, Rauws EA, Tytgat GN, Huibregtse K. Randomised trial of self-expanding metal stents versus polyethylene stents for distal malignant biliary obstruction. Lancet 1992;340(8834–8835):1488–92.

[26] Rosemurgy AS, Burnett CM, Wasselle JA. A comparison of choledochoenteric bypass and cholecystoenteric bypass in patients with biliary obstruction due to pancreatic cancer. Am Surg 1989;55(1):55–60.

[27] Sarfeh IJ, Rypins EB, Jakowatz JG, Juler GL. A prospective, randomized clinical investigation of cholecystoenterostomy and choledochoenterostomy. Am J Surg 1988; 155(3):411–4.

[28] Gentileschi P, Kini S, Gagner M. Palliative laparoscopic hepatico- and gastrojejunostomy for advanced pancreatic cancer. Journal of the Society of Laparoendoscopic Surgeons 2002; 6(4):331–8.

[29] Rothlin MA, Schob O, Weber M. Laparoscopic gastro- and hepaticojejunostomy for palliation of pancreatic cancer: a case controlled study. Surg Endosc 1999;13(11):1065–9.

[30] Nieveen van Dijkum EJ, Romijn MG, Terwee CB, de Wit LT, van der Meulen JH, Lameris HS, et al. Laparoscopic staging and subsequent palliation in patients with peripancreatic carcinoma. Ann Surg 2003;237(1):66–73.

[31] Chekan EG, Clark L, Wu J, Pappas TN, Eubanks S. Laparoscopic biliary and enteric bypass. Semin Surg Oncol 1999;16(4):313–20.

[32] Bornman PC, Harries-Jones EP, Tobias R, Van Stiegmann G, Terblanche J. Prospective controlled trial of transhepatic biliary endoprosthesis versus bypass surgery for incurable carcinoma of head of pancreas. Lancet 1986;1(8472):69–71.

[33] van den Bosch RP, van der Schelling GP, Klinkenbijl JH, Mulder PG, van Blankenstein M, Jeekel J. Guidelines for the application of surgery and endoprostheses in the palliation of obstructive jaundice in advanced cancer of the pancreas. Ann Surg 1994;219(1):18–24.

[34] Raikar GV, Melin MM, Ress A, Lettieri SZ, Poterucha JJ, Nagorney DM, et al. Cost-effective analysis of surgical palliation versus endoscopic stenting in the management of unresectable pancreatic cancer. Ann Surg Oncol 1996;3(5):470–5.

[35] Smith AC, Dowsett JF, Russell RC, Hatfield AR, Cotton PB. Randomised trial of endoscopic stenting versus surgical bypass in malignant low bile duct obstruction. Lancet 1994;344(8938):1655–60.

[36] Watanapa P, Williamson RC. Surgical palliation for pancreatic cancer: developments during the last two decades. Br J Surg 1992;79(1):8–20.

[37] Lillemoe KD, Cameron JL, Hardacre JM, Sohn TA, Sauter PK, Coleman J, et al. Is prophylactic gastrojejunostomy indicated for unresectable periampullary cancer? A prospective randomized trial. Ann Surg 1999;230(3) [discussion: 328–30]:322–8 [discussion: 77–8].

[38] Espinel J, Vivas S, Munoz F, Jorquera F, Olcoz JL. Palliative treatment of malignant obstruction of gastric outlet using an endoscopically placed enteral Wallstent. Dig Dis Sci 2001;46(11):2322–4.

[39] Lillemoe KD, Cameron JL, Kaufman HS, Yeo CJ, Pitt HA, Sauter PK. Chemical splanchnicectomy in patients with unresectable pancreatic cancer: a prospective randomized trial. Ann Surg 1993;217(5) [discussion: 456–7]:447–55 [discussion: 77–8].

[40] Gress F, Schmitt C, Sherman S, Ikenberry S, Lehman G. A prospective randomized comparison of endoscopic ultrasound- and computed tomography-guided celiac plexus block for managing chronic pancreatitis pain. Am J Gastroenterol 1999;94(4):900–5.

[41] Pietrabissa A, Vistoli F, Carobbi A, Boggi U, Bisa M, Mosca F. Thoracoscopic splanchnicectomy for pain relief in unresectable pancreatic cancer. Arch Surg 2000;135(3):332–5.

[42] Lillemoe KD, Cameron JL, Yeo CJ, Sohn TA, Nakeeb A, Sauter PK, et al. Pancreatico-duodenectomy: does it have a role in the palliation of pancreatic cancer? Ann Surg 1996;223(6) [discussion: 725–8]:718–25 [discussion: 77–8].

ELSEVIER
SAUNDERS

Surg Clin N Am 85 (2005) 373–382

SURGICAL
CLINICS OF
NORTH AMERICA

Transplantation and Palliative Care: The Convergence of Two Seemingly Opposite Realities

Ernesto P. Molmenti, MD, PhD[a],
Geoffrey P. Dunn, MD, FACS[b],*

[a]The Johns Hopkins University School of Medicine,
1830 East Monument Street, Baltimore, MD 21205, USA
[b]Department of Surgery and Palliative Care Consultation Service,
Hamot Medical Center, 201 State Street, Erie, PA 16550, USA

The concept of palliative care has rarely, if ever, been associated with transplantation. Whereas the former is considered the terminal care of irreversible disease, the latter constitutes (in the case of vital organs) the only alternative to certain death. The sharp observer, however, will realize that the concepts of palliative care and disease-directed treatment converge and coexist in the field of transplantation. This convergence is especially relevant to patients who are awaiting a transplant and patients who have inadequate allograft function.

Whether transplantation is performed for vital organs whose failure leads to death (eg, liver, heart, lung) or for organs whose failure leads to debilitating and life-limiting conditions (eg, kidney, pancreas), the diagnosis of end-stage organ failure is always present. Hand-in-hand with the disease of end-stage organ failure which can limit life occurs the experience of chronic illness which compromises quality of life.

Similar to the modern origins of hospice and palliative care [1], it was the work of a few and selected individuals that transformed transplantation from the expression of a creative idea into an ever-growing reality [2]. In addition to surgical skills, a comprehensive interdisciplinary approach is required for the adequate care of patients who have end-stage organ illness. The American Board of Surgery recently stated that surgeons should "have knowledge and skills in palliative care and management of pain, weight loss,

* Corresponding author.
E-mail address: gpdunn1@earthlink.net (G.P. Dunn).

0039-6109/05/$ - see front matter © 2005 Elsevier Inc. All rights reserved.
doi:10.1016/j.suc.2005.01.021   *surgical.theclinics.com*

and cachexia in patients with...chronic conditions" [3]. We agree with such a statement, but believe that surgeons and patients should be more familiar with palliative care, itself, as well as the unique problems of the pre- and posttransplanted state that would benefit from palliative care expertise.

Numerous examples from the history of surgery demonstrate that control of distressing symptoms and suffering never has undermined the goals of prolonging life or curing disease. Interventions that originally were designed to relieve suffering have extended life. The first successful human renal transplant by Murray in 1954 stands out as one of the most well-known modern examples of this pattern [3a].

Despite the presence of palliative medicine as an established medical specialty in the United Kingdom and the active growth of the discipline in the United States and Canada, there is scant literature or experience that directly links transplantation with palliative care. The "gold standard" of palliative medicine, *The Oxford Textbook of Palliative Medicine*, now in its third edition, has only one reference each to kidney and liver transplantation [4]. One article from the Scottish Liver Transplant Unit (Edinburgh) recommends consideration of a palliative care approach in instances of graft failure because of the increased mortality rate that is associated with retransplantation [5]. Allocation of scarce organs is directly impacted by decisions to retransplant, and these decisions are influenced by quality of life considerations, the main focus of palliative care.

It is ironic that the field of transplantation has been mostly untouched by palliative care clinicians, despite the fact that the patient population has a high age-adjusted mortality rate and virtually all suffer from chronic, progressive, and incurable illness. This is probably due to the prevailing values of a surgical culture that emphasizes salvation of life, regardless of context or consequences. In contrast to this, the words "palliation" and "palliative" are used ambivalently, even pejoratively, in the surgical literature [6].

We thought about multiple ways in which to address palliative care in transplantation. After an unproductive search of the published literature, we decided it best to use the *Statement on Principles Guiding Care at the End of Life*, that was developed by the American College of Surgeons Committee on Ethics and approved by the Board of Regents [7], as the logical choice of a conceptual framework for describing palliative care in the setting of transplantation, a surgical discipline. Our discussion is guided by their outline of principles on a point-by-point basis, while adapting them to our views on transplantation. It is hoped that the thoughts we share will plant a seed for the development of the evolving new field of palliative care in transplantation [8,9]. Our ultimate goal is to improve patient care.

Respect the dignity of the patient and caregivers

Patients who are awaiting a transplant and patients who reject allografts and their families are highly vulnerable, physically, socio-economically, psychologically, and spiritually from the consequences of end-stage organ failure. End-stage organ failure presages certain death (in the case of vital organs) or (in the case of nonvital ones) a severely compromised quality of life. The only way to prevent such outcomes is to receive a successful transplant within a brief period of time; this is a recipe for anxiety that elicits a host of coping mechanisms that are associated with it. Dignity is compromised whenever a patient or his family is overwhelmed by high physical, economic, psychologic, and existential burden; this is expressed frequently in statements such as, "I have been reduced to this" or "I can't even recognize myself." These feelings of vulnerability and impending death are fueled further by the morbidities that are associated with transplantation and immunosuppression, many of which may not be acceptable to some patients. To the transplant team, this principle is a reminder that preservation or restoration of hope is the first step in the restoration of health whatever the means. For an encephalopathic patient who is awaiting a transplant and is pulling off clothes, mumbling, and fidgeting, control of these symptoms with the effective pharmacotherapy that is available is only one of the ways in which this first principle is affirmed; there can be no sense of hope without dignity.

Be sensitive to, and respectful of, the patient's and family's wishes

Patients and their families may have different wishes that vary according to the progression of the underlying disease. The desire to proceed at any cost may be diminished as the assurance for success decreases. Such success may involve the function of the implanted organ and factors, such as neurologic recovery and expected quality of life.

Informed consent and autonomy of decision are relevant components in decision-making [10]. In addition, other variables come into play. Transplant surgeons and their patients are faced with multiple unknowns. One such situation is the need to evaluate deceased donors over a period of time that may last for less than 1 hour. The decision of whether to use a deceased donor organ is based on limited and incomplete information that is provided by the procuring agency during a telephone conversation, and without the benefit of the accepting physician performing a physical examination. In addition to the imperfect information that is provided, the accepting surgeon has to consider the imminence of death of the potential recipient (sometimes a matter of hours), and the time limits that are allowed before the organ is offered to another potential recipient on the waiting list of the same or a different institution. Although many pathologic conditions can be detected by means of such a system, many others go undetected until they manifest themselves in the recipient. Informed consent for the transplantation of such pathologies cannot be obtained because the transplanting surgeon has no knowledge of their existence. Adequate informed consent is one example of effective communication, the cardinal skill of all branches of palliative care.

Use the most appropriate measures that are consistent with the choices of the patient or the patient's legal surrogate

Transplantation introduces a new variable into the classic concepts of palliative care. The survival of a person on the waiting list is contingent upon the demise of a healthy individual or a surgical intervention that is performed in an otherwise healthy subject. Furthermore, the allocation of such organ to a recipient implies that another waiting-list patient may die as a result of the lack of an available organ.

Transplantation can provide a means of survival or a limited prolongation of life [10]. In the former case, the recipient enjoys all of the benefits of the procedure. In the latter case, as is observed in some instances of extended indications for transplantation, the benefits are associated with a limited prolongation of life [3]. It is in such cases that palliative care assumes a major role.

Other factors also should be considered. Physicians who are responsible for making the decision to proceed with transplantation may encounter certain challenges that are associated with specific patient requests. One such example is the expectation not to receive blood products during transplantation. Although reports of successful series that honored this request can be found in the transplant literature, patients and their families should be made aware of the potential risks and complications that this may entail. The surgeon also should determine whether the case can be performed under such circumstances, whether the patient would benefit from referral to a center with greater experience, the safe timing period to proceed with such intervention, and the time when the patient is no longer a candidate for transplantation under circumstances that honor his/her request.

Ensure alleviation of pain and management of other physical symptoms

Patients who have end-stage organ failure share a multitude of physical and psychologic needs that require specialized care. Being on a transplant waiting list does not diminish any of these. Patients who have received transplants and those awaiting transplant should be entitled to the same care, as long as adjunctive palliative treatment does not diminish the chances of receiving an allograft or recovery after transplantation. Moreover, there is strong theoretic plausibility and anecdotal evidence that good symptom control in nonmalignant conditions prolongs life. Patients who are not delirious are less likely to harm themselves and others; patients who have effective pain control are less likely to suffer the consequences of continuously elevated sympathetic tone and have at least one less risk factor for the development of depression. Other symptoms that are frequent in all populations who are awaiting a transplant include asthenia, nausea, cachexia, dyspnea, and pruritus. One of the strongest arguments for engaging palliative care expertise in a transplant program is to optimize control of burdensome symptoms to supplement the efforts of nursing personnel and surgeons who may have limited time and experience.

Also to be considered is the performance of invasive procedures for palliation of symptoms from end-stage organ failure, such as stenting to relieve jaundice that is due to biliary stricture or transjugular intrahepatic portosystemic shunt for intractable ascites. This type of intervention is distinct from disease (cancer) treatments, other than transplantation, that are performed to prevent mortality, regardless of the presence of symptoms. An example of this is the treatment of hepatocellular carcinoma in the setting of end-stage cirrhosis during the waiting period for transplant. Multiple studies have addressed potential treatments, or the lack of such treatments, during the waiting period [11,12]. Results differ, recommendations vary, and morbidities fluctuate. The limited availability of organs leads to the preferred treatment for those indications with the best long-term survival outcomes and the transplantation of patients who have the most advanced disease [10]. This leads, in part, to the large number of candidates that remain on waiting lists for long periods of time, until transplantation or death.

It is up to the surgeon to explain to the patient the difference between the two classes of invasive procedure, because many believe that any surgical intervention is an attempt to cure, no matter how remote or irrelevant that possibility may be. For disease-reducing treatments and symptom palliation, the ideal selection is the most effective treatment with the least morbidity and mortality. Short- and long-term results should be evaluated continuously, and adjustments should be made based on such results.

Recognize, assess, and address psychologic, social, and spiritual problems

Transplantation depends on the support of society. The experience of receiving an organ from another human being is a formidable one. Except in cases of retransplantation, it is a totally new aspect of life. Doubts, fears, goals, hopes, values, wishes, feelings of guilt, and questions inevitably surface and must be addressed. Although some problems may be common to many, others have to be answered on an individual basis. Life-limiting diseases, grief, and end-of-life issues are major topics in the minds of patients who are being considered for transplantation [13,14]. In transplantation, deaths that occur while on the waiting list should not be attributed to medical failures, but rather, mostly, to the lack of available organs [3].

Transplantation sometimes is performed in the setting of active or treated malignancies. Examples of the former include the presence of hepatocellular carcinoma and hepatoblastoma that are limited to the liver [8,9]. Examples of the latter include cases of renal cell carcinomas that are treated by removal of the involved organs, or other cancers that have shown no recurrence after a period of time that is considered to be reasonable by the treating physicians. In some cases, such malignancies may predispose to the appearance of other malignancies in the form of specific syndromes [15].

Many times, patients' expectations of a complete recovery may be unwarranted, because they may not be consistent with age, previous abilities, and comorbidities. In addition to these observations, factors (eg, previous substance abuse, infectious agents [hepatitis C]), that result from risk-taking behaviors signal significant behavioral health issues that always will remain part of a person-based assessment. Patients should receive specialized assessment and counseling to address these problems, active or not. Although a baseline functional recovery is expected in cases of successful transplantation, the range of improvement varies widely.

Ensure appropriate palliative care and hospice care

The number of patients that is on waiting lists for transplantation continues to increase at a rate that exceeds that of suitable available organs. Efforts are being made to ensure that those who have the shortest life expectancy receive the first available organs, and to diminish deaths while on the waiting lists [16,17]. Those who are transplanted have a chance to recover and to achieve a lifestyle that may allow them to enjoy life; however, those who are not fortunate enough to receive a transplant do not differ from patients who have end-stage organ failure who do not qualify for transplantation. Given the fact that there is no way to determine who will receive an organ, we believe that all patients who have end-stage organ failure should be offered palliative care consultation or hospice referral, if appropriate. Such care should not be solely comfort care, but should include keeping the option of transplantation open as long as possible while providing aggressive symptom management through close collaboration among specialists in palliative care and transplantation. A maxim that summarizes this and is heard often in palliative and hospice care is to "hope for the best and plan for the worst."

Of interest to surgeons who are comfortable with the concept of triage, is a promising model for classifying palliative care that was developed by Downing and colleagues [18]. The Victoria BGY model triages patients who are referred for palliative care according to active, comfort only, and urgent categories (see article elsewhere in this issue for more information about this topic). Active palliation (blue) encompasses investigations and treatments whose primary emphasis is control of symptoms and improved quality of life through modification of the disease process itself. The purpose of treatment is not aimed at extending life, although this may occur. Comfort only palliation (green) is reserved for patients whose demise is fairly imminent. Typically, interventions are noninvasive and rely primarily on pharmacologic treatment that does not modify the disease process. Urgent palliation (yellow) is emergent management of moderate to severe symptoms with the intention of relief within hours; it often requires medication dosages that are much greater than those which are familiar to most physicians. In cases of imminent demise, life may be shortened, although this is not the intent of treatment.

There is nothing in the Victoria BGY model that would undermine the ultimate goal of successful transplantation, and the range of palliative intervention distances palliative care from its previous negative association with "terminal" care.

For patients who have selected not to pursue the option of transplantation, hospice referral should be offered if the patient meets criteria for 6 months or less prognosis, based on the physician's or [hospice] medical director's judgment regarding the normal course of the individual's illness [19]. Some individuals may benefit from a hospice evaluation—even if they remain on a transplant list—to prepare themselves better should future circumstances not allow transplantation. The National Hospice and Palliative Care Organization (formerly the National Hospice Organization) developed prognostic criteria for patients who have nonmalignant disease to help physicians determine an individual's appropriateness for hospice care [20]. General criteria are a life-limiting condition with evidence of disease progression or impaired nutritional status that is indicated by involuntary weight loss of at least 10% of body weight in the previous 6 months, and a serum albumin that is up to 2.5 g. Disease-specific criteria, including cardiac, liver, and renal disease, are available.

Respect the patient's right to refuse treatment

In transplantation, patients usually are referred for surgical evaluation after the diagnosis of end-stage organ failure is made. As such, there is a common understanding on the parts of the patient and the surgeon that the goal of treatment is to reverse such findings by means of organ replacement. The whole process of transplantation has to be discussed by one or more members of the multi-disciplinary transplant team. Potential short- and long-term complications should be addressed.

Probably one of the most traumatic events for many people is the fact that the availability of an organ is based on the death of another human being (in deceased donors), or a risky surgical intervention with the potential for death in an otherwise healthy relative/friend/individual (in live donors). Such knowledge may be difficult to accept, and, in many occasions, requires some reflective time.

A frequent finding in large transplant programs is that the surgeon who evaluates the patient may not be the same person who performs the transplant. Such logistical problems may be hard to overcome given the large number of patients on some transplant lists, the unpredictability of how busy the service will be at any given time, and the rotating assignments among surgeons. In some cases, such as when the recipient is encephalo-pathic at the time of transplantation, s/he may not meet the surgeon until after the surgery; decisions may need to be made by a family member together with a person whom they have never met before.

Recognize the physician's responsibility to forego treatments that are futile

This is an especially relevant point in transplantation, because the cost of futility is not only a personal one for the patient, his family, and the transplant team, but is an enormous cost to a society in which donated organs are scarce. It refers to the life-saving treatment itself. Many times, the attending surgeon, together with the whole multi-disciplinary team that is caring for a patient who has end-stage organ failure, must decide when not to proceed with transplantation. This decision, made with information that usually is obtained in an ICU setting, must be made with several facts in mind.

In some instances, futility may imply that the chances of recovery are far less than the standards that are expected. A well-guided discussion about treatment options can become the occasion for patients to clarify their own wishes for treatment. If an individual who has a far advanced illness recognizes that s/he is not a transplant candidate, s/he may decide to limit life support, such as cardiopulmonary resuscitation or dialysis. The End Stage Renal Disease Work Group, in their *Report from the Field*, published a do not resuscitate protocol for dialysis patients who decide to forgo future dialysis as well other helpful suggestions for the palliative care of patients who have end-stage renal disease [21]. Much of this information, although directed to nephrology care practitioners, is useful information for trans-plant programs.

Summary

One of the authors once asked a great transplant surgeon what came to his mind when asked about palliative care. He had two answers: the first, was somewhat simplistic; the second was profound. He said that this type of service was helpful in the ICU when there was not much more to be done surgically for a patient who was dying; the second, was a story about an individual whom he had transplanted three times (who survived!) because he and his team did not want the patient and family to give up hope. The second answer is fundamentally more in keeping with the philosophy of palliative care, despite the extraordinary specific circumstances. The surgeon demonstrated ongoing presence and nonabandonment. This patient was palliated, although few surgeons could have accomplished this by doing two retransplantations! Fortunately, for the less gifted and lucky, there are many ways in which to continue a meaningful presence to an ailing or dying patient on a transplant service that do not require a transplantation procedure.

One wonders why palliative care and transplantation have not been more formally acquainted in the past given the extensive overlap of the populations served, the nature of the day-to-day problems, and the intensity of the commitment to the patient. The time is ripe for a formal mutual acquaintance between palliative care specialists and transplant teams, perhaps in the format of a work group that is similar to the work groups that promoted excellence in palliative care, such as the End Stage Renal Disease Workgroup, that were grant funded by the Robert Wood Johnson Foundation. The fields of transplantation and palliative care have a treasure trove of experience that is lacking in the other that could be exchanged profitably with a great sense of satisfaction for all.

References

[1] Schonwetter RS, editor. Hospice and palliative medicine. Core curriculum and review syllabus. American Academy of Hospice and Palliative Medicine. Dubuque (IA): Kendall/ Hunt Publishing Co.; 1999.

[2] Starzl TE, Demetris AJ. Liver transplantation: a 31-year perspective Part I. Curr Probl Surg 1990;27(2):49–116.

[3] American Board of Surgery, Inc. Booklet of information. July 2001–June 2002. Philadelphia: American Board of Surgery; 2001.

[3a] Tilney NL. Transplant: From myth to reality. New Haven: Yale University Press; 2003. p. 1–320.

[4] Doyle D, Hanks G, Cherny NI, et al, editors. Oxford textbook of palliative medicine. 3rd edition. Oxford (UK): Oxford University Press; 2004.

[5] Adam S. Palliative care for patients with a failed liver transplant. Intensive Crit Care Nurs 2000;16(6):396–402.

[6] Finlayson CA, Eisenberg BL. Palliative pelvic exenteration: patient selection and results. Oncology 1996;10(4):479–84.

[7] American College of Surgeons. Principles guiding care at end of life. Bull Am Coll Surg 1998; 83:46.

[8] Molmenti EP, Klintmalm GB. Liver transplantation in association with hepatocellular carcinoma: an update of the International Tumor Registry. Liver Transpl 2002;8(9):736–48.

[9] Molmenti EP, Wilkinson K, Molmenti H, et al. Treatment of unresectable hepatoblastoma with liver transplantation in the pediatric population. Am J Transpl 2002;2(6):535–8.

[10] Malago M, Testa G, Marcos A, et al. Ethical considerations and rationale of adult-to-adult living donor liver transplantation. Liver Transpl 2001;7(10):921–7.

[11] Fisher RA, Maroney TP, Fulcher AS, et al. Hepatocellular carcinoma: strategy for optimizing surgical resection, transplantation and palliation. Clin Transplant 2002;16(Suppl 7): 52–8.

[12] Donckier V, Van Laethem JL, Van Gansbeke D, et al. New considerations for an overall approach to treat hepatocellular carcinoma in cirrhotic patients. J Surg Oncol 2003;84(1): 36–44 [discussion 44].

[13] End of Life/Palliative Education Resource Center. Available at: http://www.eperc.mcw.edu. Accessed February 14, 2005.

[14] Center for Palliative Care at Harvard Medical School. Available at: http://www.hms.harvard.edu/cdi/pallcare.

[15] Molmenti EP, Molmenti H, Weinstein J, et al. Syndromic incidence of ovarian carcinoma after liver transplantation, with special reference to anteceding breast cancer. Dig Dis Sci 2003;48(1):187–9.

[16] Freeman RB Jr, Weisner RH, Roberts JP, et al. Improving liver allocation: MELD and PELD. Am J Transpl 2004;4(Suppl 9):114–31.

[17] United Network for Organ Sharing. Available at http://www.unos.org.

[18] Downing GM, Braithwaite DL, Wilde JM. Victoria BGY palliative care model—a new model for the 1990s. J Palliat Care 1993;9(4):26–32.

[19] Benefits Protection and Improvement Act, subtitle C, section 322, amending section 1814(a)(7) of the Social Security Act: as quoted in HCFA Program Memorandum to Intermediates and Carriers, Transmittal AB-01–09, 1/24/01.

[20] Standards and Accreditation Committee. Medical Guidelines Task Force of the National Hospice Organization. Medical guidelines for determining prognosis in selected non-cancer diseases. 2nd Edition. Arlington (VA): National Hospice Foundation; 1997.

[21] Moss AH, editor. End Stage Renal Disease Workgroup: report from the field. National Program Office, Robert Wood Johnson Foundation. 2002. Available at: www.promotingexcellence.org.

SURGICAL
CLINICS OF
NORTH AMERICA

Surg Clin N Am 85 (2005) 383–391

Educating Surgeons for the New Golden Hours: Honing the Skills of Palliative Care

Joan L. Huffman, MD, FACS[a,b,*]

[a]Department of Surgery, Temple University School of Medicine,
1801 North Broad Street, Philadelphia, PA 19122, USA
[b]Crozer-Chester Medical Center, Vivaqua Pavilion, Suite 440,
One Medical Center Boulevard, Upland, PA 19013, USA

"SURGEONS must be very careful
When they take the knife!
Underneath their fine incisions
Stirs the culprit—Life!" [1]

Oh life! Surgeons excel at life-saving resuscitations and procedures, forging ahead to beat the clock in the "golden hour." Now these stalwart gladiators must hone their skills to adapt to a different golden arena, the last ticking months, days, hours, and moments of life. Palliative care is an expanding focus for the medical community, in general, and the surgical community, in particular. For many surgeons, this is an unfamiliar concept and a huge paradigm shift, a contrast from what they believe they were or are trained to do.

Historically, the surgical perspective has been one of active, aggressive care, with the surgeon dictating the course of care to the patient. Today, surgeons must look at the other side of the same coin, and flip their perspective to the one of the patient and their needs and goals. When weighing clinical options, surgeons must consider the possibility of minimally invasive interventional radiologic or laparoscopic procedures; no intervention versus extensive traditional operations; and perhaps even no fluids or nutrition versus aggressive fluid resuscitation, hyperalimentation, or tube feedings [2]. In an age of outcomes management, new end points must be established for all patients in the continuum of life to death. Surgeons must include a

* Crozer-Chester Medical Center, Vivaqua Pavilion, Suite 440, One Medical Center Boulevard, Upland, PA 19013.
  E-mail address: lavenderdoc@comcast.net

0039-6109/05/$ - see front matter © 2005 Elsevier Inc. All rights reserved.
doi:10.1016/j.suc.2004.12.002   *surgical.theclinics.com*

sensitive plan of care for those who have chronic illnesses in long-term care, not only those who are at the end of life or actively dying. The goal must be to maintain quality of life and to relieve suffering, indeed to "do no harm."

Challenges

Multiple barriers exist to the field of surgical palliative care; deeply entrenched attitudinal concepts may be the toughest ones to conquer. Surgical culture has always defined the surgeon as the "captain of the ship" and the authoritarian decision-maker, whereas the patient is the compliant acceptor of the surgeon's goals. Yes, the surgeon must obtain informed consent; however, many times, the risks and benefits are described in such a manner that "no" is not an option to the frightened, worried patient. Some surgical colleagues are truly aghast that a patient should dictate to them what the course and limitations of care should be.

The most ingrained negative view is the one of death as a medico-surgical "failure" [3]. Surgeons strive for a "good" outcome, one that traditionally has meant a recovery from surgical intervention without any significant morbidity, and certainly life, not mortality. It is easy to forget (or avoid) our own humanity, and that the ultimate outcome of each one of us in life, is death.

Today's financial climate sets an additional hurdle to leap. Overworked surgeons struggle with reduced insurance payments while malpractice rate continue to skyrocket. As surgeons see more patients in shorter time intervals to maximize their productivity, they find little time for what many consider to be "touchy-feely" interactions with patients. Most recently, reduced work hours for residents adds insult to injury as faculty and staff find themselves taking more in-house call, working longer and longer hours.

In light of all of these obstacles, why should surgeons add one more task to our already overburdened schedule?

Directives

In the quest for excellence in surgical practice, the extent of the surgeon's educational needs continues to broaden. Initially, there were recommendations that surgeons acquire additional training in palliative care; new parameters have extended this call from suggestions to requirements.

In 1998, "Principles Guiding Care at the End of Life" were developed by the American College of Surgeons (ACS) Committee on Ethics and sanctioned by the Board of Regents. These principles provided a new set of standards of care that all surgeons must pursue (Appendix 1).

Since 2001, the American Board of Surgery (ABS) has required "the general surgeon to have knowledge and skills in palliative care and the management of pain, weight loss, and cachexia in patients with malignant and chronic conditions," as well as "sensitivity to moral and ethical issues" [4].

The certifying and credentialing examinations of the ABS currently include questions that address ethical conflicts and end-of-life situations. This emphasizes and validates the need for education in the arena of palliative care in surgery.

In July 2002, the Accreditation Council on Graduate Medical Education (ACGME) introduced general competencies for all residents in six domains: (1) practice-based learning and improvement, (2) interpersonal and communication skills, (3) professionalism, (4) system-based practice, (5) patient care, and (6) medical knowledge. From July 2002 to 2006, residency programs are expected to phase in the new requirements, and by June 2006, must have in place valid learning opportunities and dependable assessment methods of their successful implementation [5].

The scope of actual requirements for education in palliative care is continuing to enlarge. Presently, medical licensure renewal in California, Florida, and West Virginia requires continuing medical education (CME) in end-of-life or palliative care. Nevada and Texas require CME in ethics/ professional responsibility. Other states are certain to follow in this path [6].

Perhaps even more importantly, surgical clients (ie, patients and their families) are organizing and demanding a true voice in their care. Public focus groups, the national media, and the Internet are active resources for education and advocacy [7]. Surgeons owe it to themselves to be at least as well-educated as their patient populations.

The question becomes how can surgeons add these new tools to the surgical armamentarium of skills? Fortunately, there is a growing set of handy resources to fulfill the educational needs of practicing surgeons and surgeons in training.

The education process: resources and venues

Two distinct populations exist; practicing surgeons and medical student/ residents in training require the same basic information but may necessitate different approaches to win understanding and compliance. Traditional ideas may need to be reshaped carefully and new skills may need to be learned.

Surgical practice can differ extensively between academic or community settings, the operating or nonoperating surgeon, and varying areas of specialty practice. Several programs are available for use and designed to fulfill the specific needs of the practicing surgeon. A good introductory primer for the surgeon is *The Surgeon and Palliative Care* which was written by two outstanding leaders in the surgical palliative care field, Drs Dunn and Milch [8].

Other resources include surgical peers with a special interest in palliative care, journal articles, CME conferences and symposia, and websites for up-to-the-minute information and links. Some curricula address underlying philosophies, whereas others concentrate on the basic "meat and potatoes" of how to implement the skill sets.

Surgical peers

A group of interested surgeons began to meet informally. Ironically, they held their first formally-sponsored meeting the day before the national end-of-life tragedy, September, 11, 2001. This group of surgical peers was the Surgeon's Palliative Care Workgroup, a collaboration of the Promoting Excellence in End-of-Life Care Program of the Robert Wood Johnson Foundation and the American College of Surgeons [9,10]. A "Report from the Field" was published that described the cumulative accomplishment of the workgroup from their inception to their current state [11].

The workgroup continues to exist; it now is incorporated formally as a subcommittee of the ACS Division of Education—the Surgical Palliative Care (SCP) Task Force (Appendix 2). The SCP Task Force and its members are available as educational resources for interested parties [12].

Journal of the American College of Surgeons

Prefaced by the statement on "Principles Guiding Care at the End of Life," the Journal of the American College of Surgeons (JACS) began a series of articles in September 2001 on surgical palliative care (see Appendix 1). To date, 37 articles have been published. On occasion, they have been illuminated by invited commentaries. The authors, members, and associates of the SCP Workgroup/Task Force were chosen for their familiarity with the areas of palliative care and hospice. A dozen of the works were included in the JACS CME program. Topics have covered a vast scope of information: from a basic introduction to surgical palliative care, philosophy, dilemmas, and legal issues, on to communication, pain and symptom management, withdrawal of extraordinary care measures, the pros and cons of surgical or interventional options, and education and research in the field of palliative care, plus many other related topics. Links to this series of articles can be found on the JACS website [13]. An exciting addition to the forum of palliative care literature will be a forthcoming compendium of these JACS articles, highlighted by keynote addresses and commentaries.

Symposia

Eight palliative care symposia have been conducted at the ACS Clinical Congresses and Spring Meetings, from October 2000 to 2004 by the members of the surgeons SCP Workgroup/Task Force (Appendix 3). A broad range of topics has been covered to address the diverse needs of practicing surgeons. These well-attended sessions included audience participation portions and thought-provoking question and answer periods. JACS Palliative Care Series has published transcripts of the Symposia of the ACS Clinical Congresses of 2001 and 2002, and the spring 2003 session [14–17].

Preliminary planning is in process for a National Conference on Surgical Palliative Care hosted by Johns Hopkins Medical Center Department of Surgery.

Education for physicians on end of life care: The EPEC project

Education for Physicians on End of Life Care, the EPEC project, is an educational tool that is composed of a compendium of fundamental knowledge and end-of-life care skills. It can be reproduced in its entirety in a 2-day conference format or presented as a single-topic workshop (ie, for a grand rounds presentation). The package includes slides for didactic presentations, participant handbooks, and videotaped role plays of physician and patient and surrogate interactions. EPEC also sponsors a "train the trainer workshop" to increase the pool of physicians that is educated in palliative care. For those with limited block time availability, the EPEC website can be accessed and the program can be used as an online self-study tool [18].

Websites

The End of Life Physician Education Resource Center (EPERC) is a vital cache of palliative care educational materials and information that is invaluable for educators and clinicians. EPERC contains an exhaustive list of training materials, including *Fast Facts* (concise one page outlines of key clinical palliative care topics), standardized patient scenarios, and sample examination questions, plus links to multiple other palliative care resources, such as books and articles, videos, funding sources, meetings, and other training venues. The center also has created some basic "starter kits" (ie, for medical student education) to facilitate curriculum development [19].

Surgical Education and Self-Assessment Program

At the direction of Dr. Ajit Sachdeva, Director of the ACS Division of Education, the SCP Task Force has submitted questions that cover crucial components of palliative care for inclusion in the next (to be published) version of Surgical Education and Self-Assessment Program (SESAP) 12. For the first time, the area of palliative will be incorporated to supplement the educational process and to prepare surgeons further for their board certification and their life's practice. SESAP can be ordered through the ACS online or print catalog [10].

Resident and medical student education

The groundwork for education in palliative care must begin with medical students. This concept is recognized and substantiated by the Liaison Committee on Medical Education which mandates that "clinical education must include. . . ." "specific instruction in communication skills. . . .", "medical ethics and human values. . .," and "experience in palliative care, pain management, and end-of-life care" [20]. Formal curriculum and supervised bedside encounters on the surgical clerkship can provide the necessary clinical exposure. An easily adapted topic is the common situation of "breaking bad news" (eg, the diagnosis of rectal cancer) to the postoperative patient [21].

The foundation of palliative care skills that is acquired in medical school can continue to be built upon as the new doctor progresses on to residency. Within the set of the six newly-introduced ACGME General Competencies, the realms of communication and professionalism offer special opportunities for focus on palliative care education [5].

The ABS realizes that there is no routine means of providing basic curricula in a uniform format to all surgical residency programs in the United States, and as such, have committed themselves to accomplishing that goal. "The second resolution of the (ABS) January retreat supported the development of a standardized national surgery residency core curriculum. . .requirements for fulfilling the six competencies that together form the lifelong commitment to education and learning as defined by the ACGME and the American Board of Medical Specialties" [5,22].

In the interim, surgery residency directors can avail themselves of the resources of the National Residency End-of-Life Education Project that is sponsored by the Robert Wood Johnson Foundation [23]. This program was developed in 1998 by David E. Weissman, MD, Director of Palliative Care Services of the Medical College of Wisconsin, for teaching internal medicine residents. It has been expanded to include family practice, neurology, and most recently, in 2002, general surgery residents. The skill domains that are taught include: (1) communication skills, (2) ethics, (3) pain and symptom management, and (4) terminal care. To date, 30 surgical residency representatives, surgery program directors (or their designee), and chief residents have attended a "teach the teachers" format program. The charge to the attendees is to return to their home program and to incorporate the information into their own curriculum. Program faculty, with backup from the SCP Task Force, is available as resources and mentors to guide the newly-trained teachers.

Practicing surgeons who have undertaken the initiative to bolster their own palliative care education can serve as role models to their students and to their surgical colleagues in departmental meetings. Death is the ultimate outcome of all. In some specific instances, a brief palliative procedure or medical relief from symptoms to allow a quiet, comfortable death may be the preferred patient outcome, rather than an all-day commando operation, followed by months of critical care interventions, followed by the same result—death. This concept should be interwoven, where appropriate, into the traditional morbidity and mortality conference.

Summary

All surgeons should maintain a lifetime commitment to education and learning. Those who already are in practice need to make the effort to obtain or refresh their education in basic competencies in palliative care and to provide a measured balance between philosophy and practical skills.

Many resources and teaching tools are available to assist in this continuing process: surgical peers (and peers from other medical specialties), journals, textbooks, CME conferences, surgical governance and educational organizations, and palliative care websites. A tremendous summary article on palliative care education for surgeons was published recently in JACS [24].

Surgeons must be competent in the following palliative care skills: communication, holistic patient evaluation, control of pain and symptoms, understanding legal/ethical issues, withdrawing care, and the continuum of acute to chronic to terminal care. If they cannot attend to all of these areas individually, they need to be aware of the local, regional, and national resources that are available to assist the patient (or their surrogate decision maker) and themselves in the end-of-life arena. Consultations and referrals should be accomplished in such a manner that the patient does not feel abandoned by his/her surgeon at such a critical point in his/her life.

Practicing surgeons also must be involved actively in the education of resident and medical students in didactic and clinical situations. Most importantly, they must model the appropriate behaviors for their charges personally, whether it be in the consultation room breaking bad news compassionately or at the bedside easing the path to the next world. In these golden hours, the educated surgeon who wields new and mighty resources can be the greatest champion of the patient who is at the end of life.

Appendix 1: Principles guiding care at the end of life

Respect the dignity of patient and caregivers.
Be sensitive to and respectful of the patient's and family's wishes.
Use the most appropriate measures that are consistent with the choices of the patient or the patient's legal surrogate.
Ensure alleviation of pain and management of other physical symptoms.

Recognize, assess, and address psychologic, social, and spiritual problems.

Ensure appropriate continuity of care by the patient's primary or specialist physician.

Provide access to therapies that realistically may be expected to improve the patient's quality of life.

Provide access to appropriate palliative care and hospice care.

Respect the patient's right to refuse treatment.

Recognize the physician's responsibility to forego treatments that are futile.

From Bull Am Coll Surg 1998;83(4):46; with permission.

Appendix 2: Executive Group, Surgical Palliative Care Task Force, Division of Education, American College of Surgeons

Geoffrey Parker Dunn, MD, FACS, Erie, PA, Co-chair
Karen Jean Brasel, MD, FACS, Milwaukee, WI
Timothy G. Buchman, PhD, MD, St. Louis, MO
Joseph M. Civetta, MD, FACS, Farmington, CT
Alexandra M. Easson, MD, FRCS (C), Toronto, Ontario, Canada
Daniel Benjamin Hinshaw, MD, FACS, Ann Arbor, MI
Joan Lynn Huffman, MD, FAC, Upland, PA
Robert Scott Krouse, MD, Tucson, AZ
K. Francis Lee, MD, FACS, Springfield, MA
Laurence Edward McCahill, MD, FACS, Buffalo, NY
Robert Alan Milch, MD, FAC, Buffalo, NY, Co-chair
Anne Charlotte Mosenthal, MD, FACS, Newark, NJ
Albert Reed Thompson, MD, FACS, Little Rock, AR

Appendix 3: Palliative Care Symposia at the American College of Surgeons Clinical Congresses and Spring Meetings, October 2000 to October 2004

October 2000 Palliative Care by the Surgeon: Patient Selection and Management

October 2001 Palliative Care: How I Do It

April 2002 Palliative Care in Surgery

October 2002 Medical Futility and Withdrawal of Care: When Do We Stop, and How Do We Do It?

April 2003 Clinical Palliative Care in the Trenches

October 2003 Palliation as a Core Surgical Principle

April 2004 Surgical Palliation of Advanced Cancer: What's New, What's Helpful?

October 2004 Beyond Survival in Surgical Care: What the Patient Wants and What the Surgeon Should Know

April 2005 Scheduled: topic to be announced

References

[1] Dickinson E. The complete poems of Emily Dickinson. Boston: Little, Brown; 1924.

[2] Huffman JL, Dunn GP. The paradox of hydration in advanced terminal illness. J Am Coll Surg 2002;194(6):835–9.

[3] Block SD. Medical education in end-of-life care: the status of reform. J Palliat Med 2002; 5:243–8.

[4] American Board of Surgery. Available at: http://www.absurgery.org. Accessed August 30, 2004.

[5] Accreditation Council on Graduate Medical Education. Available at: http://www. acgme.org/. Accessed August 30, 2004.

[6] American Medical Association. Continuing medical education for licensure reregistration. State medical licensure and requirements and statistics 2005. Available at: http:// www.ama-assn.org/ama1/pub/upload/mm/40/tab14–05.pdf. Accessed August 30, 2004.

[7] Last acts. Available at: http://www.lastacts.org. Accessed August 30, 2004.

[8] Milch RA, Dunn GP. The surgeon and palliative care. Bull Am Coll Surg 1997;82:15–8.

[9] Robert Wood Johnson Promoting Excellence in Palliative Care. Available at: http:// www.PromotingExcellence.org. Accessed August 30, 2004.

[10] American College of Surgeons. Available at: http://facs.org/. Accessed August 30, 2004.

[11] Office of Promoting Excellence in End-of-Life Care: Surgeons' Palliative Care Workgroup Report from the Field. Palliative Care Workgroup. J Am Coll Surg 2003;197(4):661–86.

[12] The Surgical Palliative Care Task Force. Available at: http://www.facs.org/palliativecare/ index.html. Accessed August 30, 2004.

[13] Journal of the American College of Surgery. Available at: http://www.journalacs.org/. Accessed August 30, 2004.

[14] Dunn GP, Milch RA, Mosenthal AC, et al. Palliative care by the surgeon: how to do it. J Am Coll Surg 2002;194(4):509–37.

[15] Hinshaw DB, Pawlik T, Mosenthal AC, et al. When do we stop, and how do we do it? Medical futility and withdrawal of care. J Am Coll Surg 2003;196(4):621–51.

[16] Lee KF, Purcell GP, Hinshaw DB, et al. Clinical palliative care for surgeons: Part 1. J Am Coll Surg 2004;198(2):303–19.

[17] Lee KF, Johnson DL, Purcell GP, et al. Clinical palliative care for surgeons: Part 2. J Am Coll Surg 2004;198(3):477–91.

[18] The EPEC Project. Education of Physicians on End-of-Life Care. Available at: http:// www.epec.net. Accessed August 30, 2004.

[19] The End of Life Physician Education Resource Center. Available at: http://www.eperc. mcw.edu. Accessed August 30, 2004.

[20] Liaison Committee on Medical Education. Available at: http://www.lcmc.org/. Accessed August 30, 2004.

[21] Colletti L, Gruppen L, Barclay M, et al. Teaching students to break bad news. Am J Surg 2001;182:20–3.

[22] Maier RV. Report from the Chair. Am Board Surg News Summer 2004, p. 2.

[23] National Residency End-of-Life Education Project. Available at: http://www.mcw.edu/ display/router.asp?docid = 3290. Accessed August 30, 2004.

[24] Brasel KJ, Weissman DE. Palliative care education for surgeons. J Am Coll Surg 2004; 199(3):495–9.

ELSEVIER
SAUNDERS

Surg Clin N Am 85 (2005) 393–398

SURGICAL
CLINICS OF
NORTH AMERICA

Index

Note: Page numbers of article titles are in **boldface** type.

A

Acetaminophen, for chronic pain, in surgical patients, 219

α2 Adrenergic agonists, for neuropathic pain, in surgical patients, 233

Advance directives, in surgical palliative care, 276–277
    legal issues in, 292–293

Advanced cancer, **237–255**
    anorexia and cachexia in, 237–240
        assessment of, 239–240
        management of, 240
        pathophysiology of, 238–239
        quality-of-life instruments in, 239–240
    constipation in, 248–250
        assessment of, 249
        etiology of, 249
        management of, 249–250
        pathophysiology of, 248–249
    delirium in, 243–245
        diagnosis of, 243
        management of, 244–245
        pathophysiology of, 243–244
    dyspnea in, 240–242
        assessment of, 241
        management of, 241–242, 315
            anxiolytics in, 242
            bronchodilators in, 242
            opioids in, 241–242
            oxygen in, 242
            steroids in, 242
        pathophysiology of, 240–241
    fatigue in, 247–248
        assessment of, 247–248
        etiology of, 247
        management of, 248
        pathophysiology of, 247
    nausea and vomiting in, 245–247
        assessment of, 246
        etiology of, 245–246
        management of, 246–247
        pathophysiology of, 245
    resting energy expenditure in, 238

γ-Aminobutyric acid agonists, for neuropathic pain, in surgical patients, 232

Amputation, neuropathic pain after, 228

Anesthetics, local, for neuropathic pain, in surgical patients, 233

Anorexia, in advanced cancer. *See* Advanced cancer.

Antiarrhythmics, for neuropathic pain, in surgical patients, 233

Anticonvulsants, for neuropathic pain, in surgical patients, 231–232
    to prevent seizures, from brain metastases, 331

Antidepressants, for neuropathic pain, in surgical patients, 231

Anxiolytics, for dyspnea, in advanced cancer, 242

B

Baclofen, for neuropathic pain, in surgical patients, 232

Benzodiazepines, for neuropathic pain, in surgical patients, 232

Biliary cancer. *See* Pancreatic/biliary cancer.

Bisphosphonates, for impending pathologic fractures, 350

Brain metastases, **329–345**
    clinical features of, 392–393
    epidemiology of, 392–393
    management of, for multiple or recurrent metastases, 336–337
        from breast cancer, 339
        from colorectal cancer, 339
        from lung cancer, 338–339
        from melanoma, 339–340
        from prostate cancer, 340
        from renal cell carcinoma, 339